Theories and Models
in Cellular Transformation

Scientific Committee

L. Santi
Chairman

President, Italian League Against Cancer;
Director, National Institute for Cancer
Research, Genoa, Italy

S. Bergström

Chairman of the Board of Directors,
The Nobel Foundation Karolinska Institutet,
Stockholm, Sweden

L. Chieco Bianchi

Chair of Oncology, University of Padua,
Italy

G. Della Porta

Director, Laboratory of Experimental
Oncology; National Institute for Cancer
Research and Therapy, Milan, Italy

R. Dulbecco

Nobel Laureate
Salk Institute, San Diego, USA

R. Paoletti

President Foundation Lorenzini, Milan,
Italy

S. Pontremoli

Dean of the School of Medicine and Surgery,
University of Genoa;
Director, Institute of Biological Chemistry,
University of Genoa, Italy

G. Prodi

Director, Institute of Cancerology,
University of Bologna, Italy

D. Riffero

Local Committee, Celebration 150th Anni-
versary of the birth of Alfred B. Nobel
San Remo, Italy

L. Zardi

Director, Cell Biology Laboratory,
National Institute for Cancer Research,
Genoa, Italy

Theories and Models in Cellular Transformation

Edited by

L. Santi *and* Luciano Zardi

Istituto Scientifico Tumori
Genoa, Italy

1985

ACADEMIC PRESS

(*Harcourt Brace Jovanovich, Publishers*)
London   Orlando   San Diego   New York
Toronto   Montreal   Sydney   Tokyo

Academic Press Rapid Manuscript Reproduction

ACADEMIC PRESS INC. (LONDON) LTD.
24-28 Oval Road
LONDON NW1 7DX

United States Edition published by
ACADEMIC PRESS, INC.
Orlando, Florida 32887

BRITISH LIBRARY CATALOGUING IN PUBLICATION DATA
Theories and models in cellular transformation.
    1. Cancer cells
    I. Santi, L.   II. Zardi, Luciano
    616.99'407   RC269
    ISBN 0-12-619080-1

LIBRARY OF CONGRESS CATALOGING-IN-PUBLICATION DATA
Main entry under title:
Theories and models in cellular transformation
    Papers presented at the First International Conference
on Progress in Cancer Research held in San Remo, Italy,
May 5-6, 1983, organized by the Italian League against
Cancer, and others.
    Includes index.
    1. Carcinogenesis—Congresses.   2. Cell transformation
—Congresses.   3. Biological models—Congresses.
I. Santi, L.   II. Zardi, Luciano.   III. International
Conference on Progress in Cancer Research (1st : 1983 :
San Remo, Italy)   IV. Lega italiana per la lotta contro
i tumori.   [DNLM: 1. Cell Transformation, Neoplastic—
Congresses.   2. Models, Biological—Congresses.
QZ 202 T396 1983]
RC268.5.T45   1985   616.99'4071   85-11050
ISBN 0-12-619080-1 (alk. paper)
PRINTED IN THE UNITED STATES OF AMERICA

85 86 87 88   9 8 7 6 5 4 3 2 1

Contents

Contents

Contributors

ALITALO, K. Department of Virology, University of Helsinki, 00290 Helsinki 29, Finland.

BARLATI, S. Institute of Biology, University of Brescia, 25100 Brescia, Italy.

BASERGA, R. Department of Pathology, Temple University, Health Sciences Center, 3322 Broad Street, Philadelphia, Pennsylvania 19104, USA.

BERENBLUM, I. The Weizman Institute of Science, Cancer Research Unit, P.O. Box 26, Rehovot, Israel.

BIOCCA, S. Istituto di Biologia Cellulare C.N.R., Via G. Romagnosi 18A, 00100 Roma, Italy.

BLATTNER, W.A. Family Studies Section, National Cancer Institute, National Institute of Health, Bethesda, Maryland 20205, USA.

BLOBEL, G. The Rockerfeller University, 1230 York Avenue, New York, New York 10021, USA.

CALISSANO, P. Istituto di Biologia Cellulare C.N.R., Via G. Romagnosi 18A, 00100 Roma, Italy.

CATTANEO, A. Istituto di Biologia Cellulare C.N.R., Via G. Romagnosi 18A, 00100 Roma, Italy.

CLARKE, M.F. Laboratory of Tumor Cell Biology, National Cancer Institute, National Institutes of Health, Bethesda, Maryland 20205, USA.

DI LUZIO, A. Istituto di Biologia Cellulare C.N.R., Via G. Romagnosi 18A, 00100 Roma, Italy

DULBECCO, R. Salk Institute, P.O. Box 1809, San Diego, California 92112, USA.

FUDENBERG, H.H. Department of Basic and Clinical Immunology and Microbiology, Medical University of South Carolina, 171 Ashley Avenue, Charleston, South Carolina 29425, USA.

GALLO, R.C. Laboratory of Tumor Cell Biology, National Cancer Institute, National Institutes of Health, Bethesda, Maryland 20205, USA.

GILMORE, R. The Rockerfeller University, New York, New York 10021, USA.

GUO, H.G. Laboratory of Tumor Cell Biology, National Cancer Institute, National Institutes of Health, Bethesda, Maryland 20205, USA.

GUSTAFSSON, B.E. President of the Cancer Research Council, Vice President of the Swedish League against Cancer, Nobelstigtesen BOX 5232 S-10245 Stockholm, Sweden.

KESKI-OJA, J. Department of Virology, University of Helsinki, 00290 Helsinki 29, Finland.

MARKS, P.A. Memorial Sloan-Kettering Cancer Center, 1275 New York, New York 10021, USA.

MERCANTI, D. Istituto di Biologia C.N.R., Via G. Romagnosi 18A, 00100 Roma, Italy.

MINTZ, B. The Institute for Cancer Research, Fox Chase Cancer Center, Philadelphia, Pennsylvania, USA.

RAJEWSKY, M.F. Institut für Zellbiologie (Tumorforschung), Universität Essen, Hofelandstrasse 55, D-4300 Essen 1, Germany.

REITZ, M.S. Jr. Laboratory of Tumor Cell Biology, National Cancer Institute, National Institutes of Health, Bethesda, Maryland 20205, USA.

RIFKIND, R.A. Memorial Sloan-Kettering Cancer Center, 1275 New York, New York 10021, USA.

SANTI, L. Istituto Nazionale per la Ricerca sul Cancro, Viale Benedetto XV, 10, 16132 Genova, Italy.

SAXINGER, W.C. Laboratory of Tumor Cell Biology, National Cancer Institute, National Institutes of Health, Bethesda, Maryland 20205, USA.

SHEFFERY, M. Memorial Sloan-Kettering Cancer Center, 1275 New York, New York 10021, USA.

TSANG, K.Y. Department of Basic and Clinical Immunology and Microbiology, Medical University of South Carolina, Charleston, South Carolina 29425, USA.

VAHERI, A. Department of Virology, University of Helsinki, 00290 Helsinki, Finland.

WALTER, P. Department of Biochemistry and Biophysics, University of California, San Francisco, California 94143, USA.

WESTIN, E. Laboratory of Tumor Cell Biology, National Cancer Institute, National Institutes of Health, Bethesda, Maryland 20205, USA.

WONG-STAAL, F. Laboratory of Tumor Cell Biology, National Cancer Institute, National Institutes of Health, Bethesda, Maryland 20205, USA.

ZARDI, L. Cell Biology Laboratory, Istituto Nazionale per la Ricerca sul Cancro, Viale Benedetto XV, 10, 16132, Genova, Italy.

Preface

The enormous amount of new data produced each month by the
various research centres makes keeping up with the latest
findings somewhat difficult, especially in a subject as multi-
faceted as cancer-related research. This once compact field
has been divided and subdivided into more specific areas of
interest and this specialization of topic, though having provided innumerable advances, has created communication problems
between the various research sectors. Too often a symposium
or conference becomes a sounding board for experts in a highly
specialized field, providing little input into the general
scientific community.

The aim of the First International Conference on Progress
in Cancer Research was to bring together researchers from
varied sectors of the field with the intent of fostering communication and contact between investigators who would not
normally meet at more specialized meetings. The conference
also gave leading experts the opportunity to indicate the more
important directions in cancer research to a highly motivated
group of listening participants.

In this volume we present the lectures which were delivered
at the Conference last May. What we are unable to present
here and what we feel was the key to the success of this conference, is the open contact and free exchange of ideas which
took place between speakers and participants.

The First International Conference on Progress in Cancer
Research was organized by the Italian League Against Cancer
and the National Institute for Cancer Research of Genoa in
collaboration with the School of Medicine of the University
of Stockholm, the School of Medicine of the University of
Genoa and the Imperia Provincial Council.

We should like to take this opportunity to thank the
speakers, participants and all those who took part in organ-
izing the conference, especially Dr G. Lotti and La Scuola
Superiore di Oncologia e Scienze Biomediche of Genoa. In
particular we should like to thank the Nobel Foundation and
the Italian Ministries of Public Health, Education and Scientific Research for their patronage. We are also grateful to

Dr S. Bergström, Dr L. Chieco Bianchi, Dr G. Della Porta and
Dr G. Prodi for their assistance as chairmen of the various
sessions.

Lastly we express our deep gratitude to Dr R. Dulbecco,
whose support and encouragement guaranteed the success of the
conference.

Leonardo Santi

Luciano Zardi

ONCOGENES, CANCER AND DEVELOPMENT

R. Dulbecco

The Salk Institute, La Jolla, California, USA

In the last several years many important discoveries have
shown that genes present in all cells of animals, from insects
to humans, are important in the induction of cancer. They are
called "oncogenes" or cancer genes. This discovery emerged
from studies of cancer-inducing viruses. We know that after
these viruses infect cells, their genome becomes integrated
in the genome of the cell (Sambrook *et al.*, 1968). Then the
viral genes are expressed, causing the cell to become neoplastic (Oda and Dulbecco, 1968). Genetic studies showed that
this effect is due to a "transforming gene" of the virus
(Vogt, 1977). It was thought, at first, that this gene was
viral; being a gene foreign to the cells, it would upset the
working of the normal genes of the cell.

Studies with retroviruses, such as the Rous Sarcoma Virus
(RSV) showed that the transforming gene is not a viral gene:
it is a cellular gene. This was established by preparing
radioactive probes homologous to the transforming gene
(Stehelin *et al.*, 1976). Using these probes it could be
shown that the gene exists in all animals, independently of
viral infection (Spector *et al.*, 1978). The gene present in
the RSV was called *src*. When the gene was sequenced, it was
shown that it is highly conserved in different animal species.
Therefore, it performs an important function in these organisms. These discoveries have an important meaning; they open
new vistas in cancer research. We now begin to appreciate
their significance, as I will show.

In a few years other oncogenes were discovered; we now know
about twenty of them (Weiss *et al.*, 1982). They are different
from each other, but some are related and form groups. All
these genes are again present in all cells, and their sequences are conserved in animal species. Each one of these

THEORIES AND MODELS
IN CELLULAR TRANSFORMATION

oncogenes is incorporated in the genome of some retrovirus,
making it capable of inducing neoplasia. The virus is merely
a carrier of the oncogene.

An important question now arises: how can cells remain
normal if they contain an oncogene? Evidently the gene must
be inactive in these cells, and must be activated when it is
captured by a virus. The problem, therefore, is how the virus
activates the oncogene.

Studies with RSV showed that the *src* gene is transcribed
more actively when it is in the virus. The reason is that the
integrated viral genome is bordered by two sequences, the so-
called "long terminal repeats" (LTR) (Blair *et al.*, 1981),
which contain strong promoters. The genes contained in the
viral genome, including *src*, are thus expressed at a high rate.
The *src* protein is then made in large amounts. This strong
expression of the oncogene may cause its activation in some
cases. This conclusion is supported by findings with another
oncogene, *mos*, which is present in a mouse sarcoma virus. The
gene present in normal cells was cloned in a vector. The
cloned gene does not transform cells, but it does if it is
attached to an LTR (van der Hoorn *et al.*, 1982).

A different mechanism of activation has emerged after a
number of oncogenes were sequenced. The gene present in the
virus is usually somewhat different from that present in the
cells. The viral genes are often deleted at the 3'-end. One
oncogene, extracted from human bladder carcinoma cells, differs from the normal counterpart in a single base, corresponding to a single amino acid difference in the protein
(Tabin *et al.*, 1982). In many cases such altered genes are
not expressed more strongly than the normal genes, showing
that activation is caused by the structural alteration.

An interesting development in this field is that the activation of oncogenes may explain why many cancers have characteristic translocations. Well known among these translocations is the "Philadelphia chromosome" present in chronic
myeloid leukaemia. Recently, characteristic translocations
were found in lymphoid tumours such as the human Birkitt
lymphoma and mouse plasmocytomas (Klein, 1983). In all these
lymphoid tumours an oncogene (*myc*) is translocated close to an
immunoglobulin gene. In lymphatic cells an immunoglobulin
gene is built by assembling pieces from different chromosomes.
In the tumours one of these pieces becomes associated, by
translocation, with the oncogene. As a result the oncogene
is activated, probably because the gene is altered on the
translocation. The expression of the translocated oncogene
may or may not be increased.

These results are extremely interesting, but there are
dubious points. The most puzzling thing is that an oncogenic

virus carrying the *myc* gene (MC29) does not cause lymphomas. Perhaps in the lymphomas the oncogene acts in concurrence with some other factor.

I will now consider human cancers different from lymphomas. Oncogenes have been demonstrated in solid human cancers by transfecting DNA extracted from the cancers to NIH-3T3 cells (Shih *et al.*, 1979). The cells become transformed. The genes can be classified by determining which restriction endonucleases abolish transfection. In this way several interesting results were obtained. For instance all mammary cancers (Lane *et al.*, 1981), whether human or murine, contain the same oncogene; bladder cancers contain a different oncogene. Another result was obtained in chicken bursal lymphomas, in which the cellular *myc* oncogene is activated by the LTR of a retrovirus. By transfection a different oncogene was identified (Goubin *et al.*, 1983). This result raises some questions about the significance of transfection experiments and oncogene detection.

In fact there is a major difficulty in the transfection experiments: NIH-3T3 cells are susceptible to only two oncogenes, which belong to the *ras* family. This means that other oncogenes could be active within the same cancer. If so one would wonder whether the activation of the oncogene is the cause or the consequence of the neoplastic state. Measuring transcription of known oncogenes does not help much because we have seen that an oncogene can be activated even if its expression does not increase. This is an important difficulty which must be overcome.

On the basis of what has been discussed so far about oncogenes, we would expect that their action would be dominant: a single active gene should be sufficient to transform a cell. Dominance of the neoplastic state certainly occurs in hybrids between lymphocytes and myeloma cells: the hybridoma cells are neoplastic. Different results were obtained with hybrids between epithelial cancer cells and normal fibroblasts: in some cases the hybrids are not neoplastic (Stanbridge *et al.*, 1982). This result can be attributed to the differences of two cell types. Apparently the oncogene active in a certain cell type can be repressed by genes of a different cell type. This result is important, because it shows that an active oncogene can still be repressed, and that whether or not repression occurs depends on the state of differentiation of the cells. This repression perhaps explains why NIH-3T3 cells are susceptible only to *ras* oncogenes: probably NIH-3T3 genes repress other oncogenes.

It is not excluded, however, that recessive mutations may be the cause of cancer. For instance, the retinoblastoma of children is caused by such mutations (Benedict *et al.*, 1983).

Perhaps they occur in a gene which represses an oncogene.

Having discussed the properties of oncogenes we may ask what do they normally do. Recent results show that they may play an important role in development. For instance, the *fos* gene, which is present in a virus causing osteosarcoma in mice, is active in various parts of the embryo and especially in the developing bone (Müller *et al.*, 1982). These genes, therefore, may have the normal function of controlling development.

Let us consider now the products of oncogenes. The product of the *src* gene is very well known: it is an enzyme, a protein kinase, which adds phosphate residues to proteins, changing their characteristics and functions (Brugge and Erikson, 1977). This enzyme has a specificity different from that of other protein kinases, because it phosphorylates tyrosine rather than other amino acids (Hunter and Sefton, 1980). It is interesting that a similar enzyme appears in cells under the influence of substances that promote cell multiplication, like epidermal growth factor. Several other oncogenes related to *src* also specify similar kinases. Some oncogenes appear to specify cell growth factors (Todaro *et al.*, 1981), whereas two specify DNA-binding proteins (Abrams *et al.*, 1982).

The action of the *src* protein explains an important feature of transformed cells: their pleiotropism. The cells undergo several changes at the same time; these changes are the consequence of phosphorylation of different proteins. Some of these proteins are known: vinculin, a protein of the cell surface (Sefton *et al.*, 1981), and three glycolytic enzymes (Cooper *et al.*, 1983). These proteins are important in cell transformation, in which both the cell surface and regulation of glycolysis are affected. Undoubtedly other proteins are also altered, perhaps including some that control the operation of cellular genes. This could account fully for the pleiotropism of *src* transformation.

By specifying the kinase, the *src* gene causes a transformation "in parallel", because most of the effects are produced by the same protein at the same time. In other cases transformation may happen "in series", different effects being produced independently and not simultaneously by different agents; oncogenes may be among such agents. This might explain why different oncogenes are sometimes active within the same cancer cells: they may act in a serial system of transformation. It is likely that both pathways of transformation are followed in most cases. Human neoplasia seem to have an important component of serial transformation, because they evolve slowly through a succession of stages.

Pleiotropism and heterogeneity are features of all neoplasias. Cancer cells express genes that are normally inactive in the differentiated cells of the organs in which they arise. This applies to the so-called "ectopic hormones" and "onco-foetal antigens". It seems that these functions are normally expressed at some previous stage of differentiation of the cells of the organ in which the organ arises. Whether this happens by a process of dedifferentiation or because the cancer derives from cells at a more primitive state of differentiation, maintaining their characteristics, remains to be established. Reactivation of inactive genes that were expressed at an early stage of differentiation is certainly possible. For instance, it can be brought about by 5-azacytidine, which inhibits DNA methylation (Ley *et al.*, 1982). If true dedifferentiation takes place in cancer, the oncogenes may do it by bringing about demethylation. This remains to be seen.

It is well known in some systems that the action of oncogenes is strictly related to the state of differentiation of the cells. For instance, marked specificities can be seen among retroviruses that affect cells of the hematopoetic system in mice (Graf and Beng, 1978). Each virus transforms cells at one (or sometimes two) well defined stages of differentiation, and alters their differentiation potential. How further differentiation is affected depends on the virus. Some block it entirely, some allow it to proceed part way or even to completion. If oncogenes interfere with DNA methylation, they may act according to the following mechanism. The oncogenes entering a cell are exposed to differentiation by cellular enzymes. The nature of these enzymes depends on the state of methylation of the cells. In some cells the oncogene ends up being methylated and remains inactive; in other cells it stays demethylated and is active. In fact in the same cell retroviral genomes can be methylated or demethylated: they are active only if they are not methylated (Stewart *et al.*, 1982). As a counterpart, an active oncogene might affect the state of methylation of cellular genes; as a result the activity of different genes and therefore the differentiative potential of the cells, would also be altered.

These observations suggest a relationship between cancer and developmental processes. This hypothesis is supported by the induction of cancer without apparent genetic damage, perhaps by a deviation of a developmental process. An example is the induction of sarcomas in rats after implanting a solid sheet of plastic or metal under the skin (Brand, 1976). If the sheet is perforated, the tumour does not form. Another example is the formation of teratocarcinomas when embryonic cells are transferred to an adult tissue (Strickland, 1981). Is the neoplastic state in these cases caused by events similar to those that occur in development?

Development takes place by subdividing the embryo into

fields. In each field a morphogenetic substance becomes distributed according to a pattern (Gierer, 1977). Organs are formed following those patterns. If the distribution of the morphogenetic substances is altered, often there is excessive growth. These events are readily recognized by manipulating the limb buds in amphibian embryos or chick embryos. If the limb bud is amputated and replaced on its own stump (preserving the original orientation), a normal limb develops. If on the contrary the bud is rotated by 180°, two limbs are formed, one the mirror image of the other (Maden, 1980). This happens because the state of the cells clashes with the amount of morphogenetic substances to which they are exposed. The extra limb can be considered a well differentiated tumour. Abnormal limb development can also be obtained by implanting a small metal sheet.

These observations may be relevant for the formation of sarcoma after implanting a solid sheet. The hypothesis is that in the subcutaneous tissues certain cells form a weak morphogenetic field. If a wound is made, a gradient forms in the field. It induces a morphogenetic process with cell proliferation and differentiation, ending up with the formation of blood vessels and scar tissue. As the wound heals, the gradient disappears. The insertion of a solid sheet also forms a gradient by preventing equalization of the morphogenetic substance. Cell proliferation and differentiation are again stimulated, but persist. A tumour develops because in some cells the state of the gene (which are those active in the adult) clashes with the morphogenetic stimulus.

There is a similar situation when embryonic cells are placed in an adult tissue. In these cells too there is a clash between the state of the genes (consonant to an early embryo) and the morphogenetic field (adult, if any). The cells give rise to a teratocarcinoma. If the teratocarcinoma cells are placed back into an early embryo they restart normal development because the genes and the field are in accord. The implanted cells differentiate normally (Illmensee and Mintz, 1976). The teratocarcinoma cells can also differentiate in culture, probably when they can reestablish some suitable morphogenetic field.

This hypothesis can also be expressed in a different way: cancer arises when certain cellular genes are subtracted from normal regulatory influences provided by the environment. This may happen because the genes are expressed in an inappropriate way, or because the normal regulatory substances are absent or are replaced by abnormal ones. In either case cellular genes are expressed in an anomalous way. The process has evolutionary capacity because the abnormal gene products may cause perturbation of the expression of additional genes, generating a cascade of events (Dulbecco, 1982). The cells may at first undergo abnormal proliferation; they may express unusual functions without becoming neoplastic. The neoplastic transformation will occur later, when the cascade leads to the activation of an appropriate oncogene.

There are other parallels between cancer and development. Both evolve through a series of stages; both are autocatalytic. In the fields of a slime mould autocatalysis is maintained by the pulsating release of cyclic AMP when a cell is stimulated by cAMP, which is the morphogenetic substance of that field (Kassin, 1981). In cancers, autocatalysis is maintained, in some cases, when the cancer cells produce growth factors that stimulate the growth of the cells themselves. It is likely also that autocatalysis occurs at the level of gene regulation and is maintained by the cascade process.

These considerations call for a reevaluation of the role of DNA alteration in cancer. Undoubtedly many carcinogens are also mutagens, but some are not (e.g., plastic sheets, asbestos, hormones). New DNA alterations, therefore, are not required for cancer induction. Chemical carcinogens do not simply alter DNA, but also RNA and proteins (Miller and Miller, 1971). Through these changes they can alter gene regulation. Substances that only alter DNA information but not other cellular macromolecules (such as 5-bromo deoxyuridine) are not carcinogens (Poirier and de Serres, 1979). It is likely that the mechanism of chemical carcinogenesis is multiple. They may change the regulation of genes by altering the DNA of control genes, or regulatory RNAs and proteins. Other substances may act by directly altering gene regulation (hormones, asbestos), or by modifying the external regulators (plastic sheets). The only requirement is that ultimately an oncogene be activated.

In conclusion, the discovery of oncogenes has revolutionized the study of cancer. The role of oncogenes suggests that cancer is the result of developmental events which take place when the state of the cellular genes clashes with that of the external morphogenetic substances. The discovery of the function of the *src* gene has opened new horizons. In part this is because enzymes with similar specificity participate in normal growth control, and perhaps mediate certain events in development.

Recognizing a relationship between cancer and development has several consequences. It encourages us to study development and its molecular mechanisms. In doing so we can take advantage of new technical tools, such as monoclonal antibodies. This approach makes us think of development when we study cancer, and invites us to use results obtained in one field in order to facilitate progress in the other field.

Morphogenetic substances which determine specific developmental stages may also play a role in cancer induction, either promoting or inhibiting it. Their identification may help us in cancer prevention or therapy. They may be capable of restoring the normal state in the neoplastic cells. Finally recognizing the relationship between the two processes may contribute to bringing cancer in line with normal biological processes.

REFERENCES

Abrams, H.D., Rohrschneider, L.R. and Eisenman, R.N. (1982). *Cell* 29, 427-439.

Benedict, W.F., Murphree, A.L., Banerjee, A., *et al.*(1983). *Science* 219, 973-975.

Blair, D.G., Oskarsson, M., Wood, T.G. *et al.* (1981). *Science* 212, 941.

Brand, K.G. (1976). *J. Natl. Cancer Inst.* 57, 973-976.

Brugge, J.S. and Erikson, R.L. (1977). *Nature (London)* 269. 346-348.

Cooper, J.,Reiss, N.A., Schwartz, R.J. and Hunter,T. (1983). *Nature (London)* 302, 218-223.

Dulbecco, R. (1982). *Endeavour*, Vol.6, 2, 59-65.

Gierer, A. (1977). *Current Topics in Development Biology* Vol. 11, 17-59.

Goubin, G., Goldman, D.S., Luce, J. *et al.* (1983). *Nature* 302, 114-119.

Graf, T. and Beng, H. (1978). *Biochim. Biophys. Acta* 516, 269-299.

Hunter, T. and Sefton, B.M. (1980). *Proc. Natl. Acad. Sci. USA* 77, 1311-1315.

Illmensee, K. and Mintz, B. (1976). *Proc. Natl. Acad. Sci. USA* 73, 549-553.

Kassin, R.H. (1981). *Cell* 27, 241-243.

Klein, G. (1983). *Cell* 32, 311-315.

Lane, M.A., Sainten, A. and Cooper, G. (1981). *Proc. Natl. Acad. Sci. USA* 78, 5185-5189.

Ley, T.J., De Simone, J., Anagnou, N.P. *et al.* (1982). *New Engl. J. Med.* 307, 1469-1476.

Maden, M. (1980). *J. Embryol. Exp. Morphol.* 56, 201-209.

Miller, E.C. and Miller, J.A. (1971). *In* "Chemical Mutagens". (Ed. A. Hollander) Vol. I, pp.83-119, Plenum Publ. Co., New York.

Müller, R., Slamon, D.J., Tremblay, J.M. *et al.* (1982). *Nature (London)* 299, 640-644.

Oda, K. and Dulbecco, R. (1968). *Proc. Natl. Acad. Sci. USA* 60, 525-532.

Poirier, L.A. and de Serres, F.J. (1979). *J. Natl. Cancer Inst.* 62, 919-926.

Sambrook, J., Westphal, H., Strinivasan, P.R. and Dulbecco, R. (1968). *Proc. Natl. Acad. Sci. USA* 60, 1288-1295.

Sefton, B.M. and Hunter, T. (1981). *Cell* 24, 165-174.

Shih, C., Shilo. B.-Z., Goldfarb, M.P. *et al.* (1979). *Proc. Natl. Acad. Sci. USA* 76, 5714-5718.

Spector, D., Varmus, H.E. and Bishop, J.M. (1978). *Proc. Natl. Acad. Sci. USA* 75, 4102-4106.

Stanbridge, E.J., Der, C.J., Doersen, C.-J. *et al.* (1982) *Science* 215, 252-259.

Stehelin, D., Varmus, H.E., Bishop, J.M. and Vogt, P. (1976). *Nature (London)* 260, 170-173.

Stewart, C.L., Stuhlmann, H., Jähner, D. and Jaenish, R. (1982) *Proc. Natl. Acad. Sci. USA* 79, 4098-4102.

Strickland, S. (1981). *Cell* 24, 277-278.

Tabin, C.T., Bradley, S.M., Borgmann, C.I. and Weinberg, R.A. (1982). *Nature (London)* 300, 143-151.

Todaro, G.J., DeLarco, J.E., Fryling, C. *et al.* (1981). *J. Supramol. Struct. and Cell Biochem.* 15, 287-301.

van der Hoorn, A., Hulsebos, E., Berns, A.J.M. and Bloemers, H.P.J. (1982). *The EMBO J.* 1, 1313-1317.

Vogt, P.K. (1977). *In* "Comprehensive Virology". (Eds. H. Fraenkel-Conrat and R. Wagner) The genetics of RNA tumor viruses, pp.341-455. Plenum Publishing Corp., New York.

Weiss, R., Teich, N., Varmus, H. and Coffin, Jr. (1982). "RNA Tumor Viruses". Cold Spring Harbor Laboratory, New York.

MOLECULAR BIOLOGY OF CELL PROLIFERATION

R. Baserga

Department of Pathology and Fels Research Institute,
Temple University School of Medicine,
Philadelphia, Pennsylvania, USA

INTRODUCTION

The two fundamental characteristics of a living cell are metabolism and reproduction. The mechanisms by which a cell divides and populations of cells grow in number are therefore of the utmost importance, above and beyond their role in abnormal growth, and our goal is to modify and correct any abnormality of cell proliferation.

This paper deals with some basic aspects of cell reproduction, and, more precisely, of cell reproduction in mammalian cells. Cell reproduction or division (the two terms can be used interchangeably) can be studied at two different basic levels: cellular and molecular. At the cellular level one studies the kinetics of populations of cells, i.e. how a population of cells reaches its optimal number and the conditions that can alter it. At the molecular level, which is the subject of this paper, we investigate the genes and the gene products that regulate cell proliferation. I will limit myself to the genes and gene products that regulate cell proliferation inside the cell, leaving to others the task of evaluating the very important field of growth stimulatory and inhibitory factors, i.e. the substances that regulate cell proliferation from outside the cells. A reasonably up-to-date review of these substances can be found in a recent book (Baserga, 1981).

MOLECULAR BIOLOGY

Every six months we witness the discovery of a new cellular component that "controls" cell proliferation. The list is

THEORIES AND MODELS
IN CELLULAR TRANSFORMATION

endless: membrane glycoproteins, membrane glycolipids, cyclic
AMP, cyclic GMP, plasminogen activator, ribosomal RNA, ornithine decarboxylase, cell size, nuclear size, Ca^{2+}, Mg^{2+},
deoxynucleotide pools, levels of thymidine kinase, histone
phosphorylation, histone dephosphorylation, phosphorylation
of non-histone proteins, and so on. The problem here is how
to define the term "control of cell proliferation". Clearly,
a cell deficient in Mg^{2+} may have trouble in carrying out some
enzymatic reactions necessary for the metabolism and reproduction of the cell. But that is not to say that Mg^{2+} levels
control the extent of cell proliferation in tissues. The con-
fusion here is between cellular components that are necessary
for cell division and those that initiate the series of processes leading to mitosis. Many genes, gene products and
other cellular components are required for a resting cell to
re-enter the cell cycle, but by "control of cell proliferation"
one should refer to the actual gene (or at the most a few
genes) that initiate the transition from a resting to a growing stage. The analogy we could make is that of a boat travel-
ling from A to B on a river with several locks. Each lock
must operate properly for the boat to arrive at its destination,
but the decision to go from A to B is made at the beginning by
the Captain, or his employers. No one has yet identified genes
or gene products (unless viral) that will trigger cells into
the cycle, but the techniques to do it are now available and
the time is not far away when these genes will be identified.
In the next few pages I will discuss what is known about the
genes and gene products that are required for cell proliferation.

Growth in Size and Cell DNA Replication

A prerequisite for cell division is an increase in size of
the cell. During balanced growth under physiological conditions: "The two daughter cells produced at each division
are identical to the parent at the same time in the preceding
cycle: this requires that all cell components are doubled
during the course of each cell cycle" (Fraser and Nurse,
1978). This is true of bacteria, yeasts (Mitchison, 1971),
and mammalian cells (Becker *et al.*, 1971; Cohen and Studzinski,
1976; Darzynkiewicz *et al.*, 1979). If the reproduction of
ribosomes is inhibited cells cannot divide, although they
enter S phase (Mora *et al.*, 1980). Similarly, the coupling
time of cells in culture is strictly dependent on the doubling time of the amount of proteins. Yet cells can enter S
phase even with subnormal amounts of proteins Rønning *et al.*,
1981). This means that growth in size and cell division
cannot be dissociated, but growth in size and cell DNA

replication can.

This conclusion has been rigorously confirmed with ts mutants of the cell cycle (see below) and with certain small DNA oncogenic viruses, such as SV40 and Adenovirus. Infection with Adenovirus 2 (or 5) causes cell DNA replication in quiescent cells in culture (Rossini *et al.*, 1979) without a concomitant increase in cell size (Pochron *et al.*, 1980). This means that the Adenovirus genome encodes information necessary and sufficient for the induction of cell DNA synthesis, but not for a doubling of other cellular components.

Even more interesting are the results obtained by direct microinjection into the nuclei of mammalian cells of fragments of SV40 genome cloned in plasmid pBR322. Using this technique of gene transfer it was possible to show that the information for cell DNA replication and for growth in size resides in two different domains of the SV40 A gene (Soprano *et al.*, 1980; Galanti *et al.*, 1981). The information for cell DNA replication can be localized to a genomic fragment of about 150 base pairs in the 5' third of the gene, while the information for growth in size is further downstream, about 300 base pairs away. The presence of two separate pieces of information on the same gene (and therefore on the same gene product) should not be surprising. It is becoming increasingly clear that many proteins are multifunctional, with different domains being critical for different functions. The SV40 A gene is not different and it encodes for a protein, the large T antigen, that has several distinct functions localizable to different domains (see the discussion in the paper by Soprano *et al.*, 1980).

Thus, it is possible to construct genes that stimulate <u>only</u> cell DNA replication or <u>only</u> growth in size. One can say that at a molecular level there are two cell cycles: one that controls cell DNA replication and one that regulates growth in size as predicted by Mitchison (1971). The two converge to produce mitosis.

Temperature-Sensitive Mutants of the Cell Cycle

It has been possible, in the past few years, to surmise the existence of genes whose expression is required for the transition of cells from G_o, or mitosis, to S. This has come about through the isolation of cell-cycle specific ts mutants, operationally defined as mutants that arrest at the non-permissive temperature in a specific phase of the cell cycle. Several such mutants have been reported and some of them are listed in Table 1. Some mutants arrest in G_1, some in S phase, others in G_2 or mitosis. Each of them is presumably defective in a gene that is required for the progression of cells

TABLE 1

Conditional Mutants of the Cell Cycle

Cell Line		Apparent Lesion	References
Chinese hamster WG-1A (K12)		late G_1	Roscoe *et al.*, '73
Syrian hamster BHK21	(tsAF8)	G_1	Burstin *et al.*, '74
	(ts13)	G_1	Talavera & Basilico '77
	(tsHJ4)	G_1	Talavera & Basilico '77
	(dna-tsBN2)	DNA synthesis	Eilen *et al.*, '80
Chinese hamster CCL39	(BF113)	G_1	Scheffler & Buttin '73
Mouse B54		G_1	Liskay '74
Hamster HM-1 (ts546)		mitosis	Wang '74
Murine leukaemia L5178Y		mitosis & cytokinesis	Shiomi & Sato '76
Chinese hamster CHO (CS4-D3)		G_1 (cold sensitive)	Crane & Thomas '76
Mouse L (tsA169)		DNA replication	Sheinin '76
Mouse Balb/3T3 (ts-2)		DNA synthesis	Slater & Ozer '76
Mouse FM3A (ts85)		late S/G_2	Yasuda *et al.*, '81
Chinese hamster WG1A (H.3,5)		G_1	Landy-Otsuka & Scheffler '80
Syrian hamster BHK21 (tsBN75)		G_2 and S	Nishimoto *et al.*, '80
Mouse FM3A (tsT244)		DNA synthesis	Tsai *et al.*, '79
Syrian hamster BHK21 (ts422E)		cell division	Mora *et al.*, '80

through that particular phase of the cell cycle. The importance of cell cyclic-specific ts mutants cannot be overestimated.
Regardless of one's view of the cell cycle, these conditional
mutants constitute a catalogue of genes whose expression is
necessary for cell proliferation. Indeed, now that gene
cloning allows the isolation and identification of genes, it
is to be hoped that other mutants can be added to those listed
in Table 1. Analysis of these mutants by recombinant DNA
technology should be very helpful in elucidating the genetic
basis of cell proliferation.

The Role of RNA Polymerase II in Cell Growth

A number of ts cell cycle mutants have been characterized at
the molecular level. For instance, the mutant described by
Tsai *et al.* (1979) is defective in DNA polymerase α. Yasuda
et al. (1981) have described a mutant of the cell cycle, ts85,
which is defective in chromosome condensation and whose defect
is related to the phosphorylation of histone H1. Another ts
mutant of the cell cycle, tsAF8 which arrests in G_1 at the
nonpermissive temperature, has been identified as a mutant of
RNA polymerase II. The characterization of this mutant began
when Rossini and Baserga (1978) showed that in tsAF8 cells the
RNA polymerase II activity of isolated nuclei disappeared with
a half-life of 10-12 h when the cells were shifted to the nonpermissive temperature. In subsequent experiments, Rossini
et al. (1980) showed that the RNA polymerase II molecule
actually disappeared with a half-life of 10-12 h when tsAF8
cells were shifted to the nonpermissive temperature. RNA
polymerase I activity was not affected and the cells remained
viable for at least 60 h although RNA polymerase I activity
was virtually gone by 24 h. A rapid survey of protein synthesis is not affected for at least 30 h at the nonpermissive
temperature (Rossini *et al.*, 1980). Furthermore, studies by
flow cytophotometry have demonstrated that tsAF8 accumulate
RNA just as effectively at the nonpermissive temperature as
at the permissive temperature (Ashihara *et al.*, 1978). Thus,
in the absence of RNA polymerase II, the cells cannot enter
S phase but they continue to symthesize rRNA and proteins at
normal rates. The final confirmation of the nature of the ts
defect came when Waechter *et al.* (unpublished data from our
laboratory) corrected the ts defect of tsAF8 cells by microinjecting them with highly purified preparations of RNA polymerase II.

   The implications of these findings are 1) RNA polymerase
II is needed for the progression of cells in G_1 which, in turn,
indicates that unique copy genes must be transcribed for entry
into S either from G_o or from mitosis; 2) while RNA polymerase

II is necessary for the entry into S, it is not required for
growth in size (as measured by the accumulation of RNA proteins); and therefore, 3) the two processes, cell DNA replication and growth in size, can again be dissociated.

Another cell cycle ts mutant, whose lesion is known, is
422E, derived, like tsAF8 and ts13, from BHK cells. This
mutant is defective in the processing of 28S ribosomal RNA
(Toniolo *et al.*, 1973). As would be expected 422E cells
enter S even at the nonpermissive temperature (Mora *et al.*,
1980), indicating that accumulation of rRNA is not necessary
for entry into S. However, at the nonpermissive temperature
422E cells do not divide, indicating a requirement for rRNA
accumulation for cell division (Mora *et al.*, 1980).

Viral Genes that Control Cell Proliferation

It has been known for several years that small DNA viruses
such as SV40, polyoma and Adenoviruses can induce resting
cells to enter the S phase (for a review see Weil, 1978). A
virus like SV40 is known under appropriate conditions to induce not only cell DNA replication, but also growth in size
of the cell and, eventually, mitosis and for this reason Weil
(1978) has called these viruses mitogenic viruses. Indeed,
the gene products of these viruses fulfill the criteria for
our definition of genes controlling cell proliferation. They
can induce cell DNA replication and division in cells that
otherwise would remain quiescent. Unfortunately, they are
viral and not cellular products. Because these viruses are
known to alter the extracellular growth requirements of normal
mammalian cells we thought it would be interesting to determine whether the information contained in the genome of some
of these viruses could also alter the requirements for certain
cellular functions necessary for the serum stimulated transition of cells from G_o to S, i.e. from a resting to a growing
stage. Thus far we have tested two DNA viruses, i.e. SV40
and Adenovirus 2.

Our results indicate that both SV40 and Adenovirus could
induce cell DNA synthesis in G_1-specific cell cycle mutants
(ts13, tsAF8) even at the nonpermissive temperatures (Rossini
et al., 1979; Floros *et al.*, 1981). More recently Kawasaki
et al. (1981) showed that SV40 can induce cell DNA synthesis
in cells exposed to concentrations of butyrate that inhibit
serum-stimulated DNA synthesis.

We can conclude from these experiments that SV40 and
Adenovirus can induce cell DNA replication in the absence of
certain intracellular gene products that are required by
serum-stimulated cells. These results explain transformation
as a mechanism by which chemically, or virally modified genes,

alter the extra- and intra-cellular growth requirements of a cell, thus conferring on it a selective growth advantage. Incidentally, these results also indicate that some genes "required" for cell proliferation can be dispensed with if the cell receives the proper amount of information.

CELL REPRODUCTION AND CELL DIFFERENTIATION

Contrary to popular belief cell proliferation and cell differentiation are not mutually exclusive. Bone marrow cells, hepatocytes, salivary gland cells, etc. are illustrations of cells and tissues in which differentiated functions can proceed *pari passu* with cell proliferation. It is true, though, that terminally differentiated cells (for instance, keratinized cells, polymorpho-nuclear leukocytes) are not capable of dividing.

One of the popular theories of cancer states that cancer is a disease of differentiation, more precisely, of blocked differentiation. As the theory goes a cancer cell is a cell that, having failed to differentiate, is locked into a proliferative stage. Clearly, one can take this statement and turn it around to read that a cancer cell is a cell in which failure of growth control causes the cell to continuously divide and, therefore, to avoid differentiation.

These theories, like the amboceptor theory of Ehrlich, were interesting and stimulating many years ago. By now they have become a semantic ploy, somewhat obsolete in a world where genes can be isolated, cut into pieces, rejoined, manufactured to order and re-introduced into other cells. Personally, I think we should enter the 20th century a few years before it ends. The recent experiments by Weinberg (Shih *et. al.*, 1981; Murray *et al.*, 1981) and Cooper *et al.* (1980) clearly show that cells in culture can be transformed by the introduction into them of genes from chemically transformed, malignant cells. Their experiments unequivocally show that some genes from tumour cells can confer on untransformed cells in culture the ability to grow indefinitely with the characteristics of malignant cells.

This is actually good news. If tumour cells have oncogenes (and dominant, at that) it may be possible to do something about them. If transformation were due to the <u>absence</u> of something it could be a hopeless situation since how can one do something against nothing? The discovery of positive effectors in the form of oncogenes could mark the beginning of a revolutionary approach to cancer therapy.

MOLECULAR TARGETS OF CANCER THERAPY

I would like now to point out certain recent advances in basic
techniques that open the way for radically new approaches to
therapy.

One approach of course is to develop weapons directed
against the oncogenes mentioned above. The way there is not
yet clear, but two other approaches are already at the stage
of feasibility: monoclonal antibodies and gene transfer.
Since this paper deals with the molecular biology of cell proliferation I will limit myself here to gene transfer. The
technique of gene transfer has unlimited possibilities in the
biological field. Basically, it consists of the phenotypic
or genotypic modification of a cell (or cells) by the introduction into it of a modifying gene. Certain viruses have
been doing this all along and, indeed, transformation by DNA
oncogenic viruses or by retroviruses consists of the integration into the cellular genome of viral genes that confer to
the cells growth advantages. But now any gene can be introduced into viable mammalian cells, there to be expressed and
to cause either phenotypic or genotypic changes, or both.
Two techniques are particularly powerful at the present time:
manual microinjection and transfection.

Manual Microinjection

With this technique, developed by several investigators and
perfected in 1976 by Graessmann and Graessmann, one can inject
directly into the nuclei of mammalian cells $\sim 5 \times ^-10^{11}$ of a
solution containing either DNA (Floros et al., 1981), mRNA
(Floros et al., 1981; Richardson et al., 1980) or proteins
(Feramisco, 1979). A good operator can inject about 400 cells
in one hour, and the efficiency with DNA is very high. In a
variety of cell lines we have been able to obtain phenotypic
efficiences of almost 100%, i.e. > 95% of the microinjected
cells expressed the product of the microinjected gene (T antigen in cells microinjected with the SV40 A gene, viral thymidine kinase in cells microinjected with the TK gene of Herpes
Simplex virus etc.). Genotypic transformation, for instance,
transformation by the SV40 A gene, can be as high as 30%
(unpublished results from our laboratory). Manual microinjection is exceedingly useful if one wishes to introduce new
genes into precisely targeted cells. It is still unrivalled,
if one wishes to introduce mRNAs or proteins.

Transfection

This procedure was developed by Graham et al. (1974) and subsequently perfected in several laboratories (Wigler et al.,

1978; Galanti *et al.*, 1981). It consists of exposing cells
to a precipitate of DNA in a solution of calcium phosphate.
Although some of the steps of DNA transfection seem straight
out of a book on magic, the technique actually works. Using
tk-ts13 cells and transfection in suspension, we have actually
been able to transfect as many as 60% of the cells in the
population, i.e. 60% of the cells expressed the product of
the transfected gene.

This is a powerful technique for transferring genes in bulk
to other cells. Transfected cells can then be selected by
using conditions that are nonpermissive except for the cells
carrying the transfected gene.

Applications

The strategy here is to protect the vulnerable tissues of the
animal body, for instance the bone marrow, by transfecting
into the cell genes that can confer to marrow cells resistance
to drugs to be used for chemotherapy. This has already been
done by Cline *et al.* (1980) who introduced DNA from a methotrexate resistant cell line into mouse bone marrow cells and
injected the treated cells into recipient mice. When the
recipient mice were treated with methotrexate, methotrexate-
resistant cells grew out to become a majority of the bone
marrow cells.

Genes for resistance to other drugs can similarly be transferred for protection of bone marrow cells. The rapid advances
in gene cloning make it likely that other genes for drug resistance will be cloned and become candidates for transfection
experiments. Indeed, one can even fantasize that *E. coli*
carrying the desired recombinant plasmids could be introduced
into the gastro-intestinal tract of animals in an attempt to
transfect the epithelial cells of the bowel that are the
second most vulnerable tissue in the body.

Although these experiments still need to be worked out
first in animals, their feasibility is self-evident. While
using the presently available anti-cancer agents, the clini-
cian should start looking forward to a time when the therapy
of cancer will be based on the explosive techniques of molecular biology.

REFERENCES

Ashihara, T., Traganos, F., Baserga, R. and Darzynkiewz, Z.
    (1978). *Cancer Res.* 38, 2514-2518.
Baserga, R. (1981). (Ed.) "Tissue Growth Factors". Vol.57
    pp.630, Springer-Verlag, Berlin.
Becker, H., Stanners, C.P. and Kudlow, J.E. (1971). *J. Cell.*

Physiol. 77, 43-50.

Burstin, S.J., Meiss, H.K. and Basilico, C. (1974). *J. Cell. Physiol.* 84, 397-408.

Cline, M.J., Stang, H., Mercola, K., Morse, L., Ruprecht, R., Broune, J. and Salser, W. (1980). *Nature* 284, 422-425.

Cohen, L.S. and Studzinski, G.P. (1976). *J. Cell. Physiol.* 69, 331-340.

Cooper, G.M., Okenquist, S. and Silverman, L. (1980). *Nature* 284, 418-421.

Crane, M. St.J. and Thomas, D.B. (1976). *Nature* 261, 205-208.

Darzynkiewicz, Z., Evenson, D.P., Staiano-Coico, L., Sharpless, T.K. and Melamed, M.L. (1979). *J. Cell. Physiol.* 100, 425-438.

Eilen, E., Hand, R. and Basilico, C. (1980). *J. Cell. Physiol.* 105, 259-266.

Feramisco, J.R. (1979). *Proc. Natl. Acad. Sci.* 76, 3967-3971.

Floros, J., Jonak, G., Galanti, N. and Baserga, R. (1981). *Exp. Cell Res.* 132, 215-223.

Fraser, R.S.S. and Nurse, P. (1978). *Nature* 271, 726-730.

Galanti, N., Jonak, G.J., Soprano, K.J., Floros, J., Kaczmarek, L., Weissmann, S., Reddy, V.B., Tilghman, S.M. and Baserga, R. (1981). *J. Biol. Chem.* 256, 6469-6474.

Graessmann, M. and Graessmann, A. (1976). *Proc. Natl. Acad. Sci.* 73, 366-370.

Graham, F.L., van der Eb, A.J. and Heikneker, H.L. (1974). *Nature* 251, 687-691.

Kawasaki, S., Diamond, L. and Baserga, R. (1981). *Mol. and Cell. Biol.* 1, 1038-1047.

Landy-Otsuka, F. and Scheffler, I. (1980). *J. Cell. Physiol.* 105, 209-220.

Liskay, R.M. (1974). *J. Cell. Physiol.* 84, 49-56.

Mitchison, J.M. (1971). "The Biology of the Cell Cycle". Cambridge University Press, London.

Mora, M., Darzynkiewicz, A. and Baserga, R. (1980). *Exp. Cell Res.* 125, 241-249.

Murray, M.J., Shilo, B.Z., Shih, C., Cowing, D. Hsu, H.W. and Weinberg, R.A. (1981). *Cell* 25, 355-361.

Nishimoto, T., Takahashi, T. and Basilico, C. (1980). *Somatic Cell Genet.* 6, 465-476.

Pochron, S., Rossini, M., Darzynkiewicz, Z., Traganos, F. and Baserga, R. (1980). *J. Biol. Chem.* 255, 4411-4413.

Richardson, W.D., Carter, B.J. and Westphal, H. (1980). *Proc. Natl. Acad. Sci.* 77, 931-935.

Rønning, Ø.W., Lindmo, T., Pettersen, E.O. and Seglen, P.O. (1981). *J. Cell. Physiol.* 109, 411-418.

Roscoe, D.H., Robinson, H. and Carbonell, A.W. (1973). *J. Cell. Physiol.* 82, 333-338.

Rossini, M. and Baserga, R. (1978). *Biochemistry* 17, 858-863.

Rossini, M., Baserga, S., Huang, C.H., Ingles, C.J. and
  Baserga, R. (1980). *J. Cell. Physiol.* 103, 97-103.
Rossini, M., Weinmann, R. and Baserga, R. (1979). *Proc. Natl.
  Acad. Sci.* 76, 4441-4445.
Scheffler, I.E. and Buttin, G. (1973). *J. Cell. Physiol.* 81,
  199-216.
Sheinin, R. (1976). *Cell* 7, 49-57.
Shih, C., Padhy, L.C., Murray, M.J. and Weinberg, R.A. (1981).
  Nature 290, 261-264.
Shiomi, T. and Sato, K. (1976). *Exp. Cell Res.* 100, 297-302.
Slater, M.L. and Ozer, H.L. (1976). *Cell* 7, 289-295.
Soprano, K.J., Rossini, M., Croce, C. and Baserga, R. (1980).
  Virology 102, 317-326.
Talavera, A. and Basilico, C. (1977). *J. Cell. Physiol.* 92,
  425-436.
Toniolo, D., Meiss, H.K. and Basilico, C. (1973). *Proc. Natl.
  Acad. Sci.* 70, 1273-1277.
Tsai, Y., Hanaoka, F., Nakano, M.M. and Yamada, M. (1979).
  Biochem. Biophys. Res. Comm. 91, 1190-1195.
Wang, R.J. (1974). *Nature* 248, 76-78.
Weil, R. (1978). *Biochem. Biophys. Acta* 516, 301-388.
Wigler, M., Pellicer, A., Silverstein, S. and Axel, R. (1978).
  Cell 14, 725-731.
Yasuda, H., Matsumoto, Y., Mita, S., Marunouchi, T. and
  Yamada, M. (1981). *Biochemistry* 20, 4414-4419.

IN UTERO OSTEOSARCOMA TOLERIZED HAMSTERS: A MODEL FOR HUMAN CANCER AND IMMUNOCYTE DIFFERENTIATION

H.H. Fudenberg and K.Y. Tsang

Department of Basic and Clinical Immunology and Microbiology, Medical University of South Carolina, Charleston, South Carolina 29425, USA

INTRODUCTION

Osteosarcoma (OS) is a malignancy that occurs primarily during the second decade of life (Dahlin and Coventry, 1967). At present there is no known mode of successful long-term therapy. Several reports have indicated that new forms of adjuvant chemotherapy can delay the occurrence of histologically evident metastases and clinical relapse (Cortes *et al.*, 1978; Jaffe *et al.*, 1978; Sutow *et al.*, 1976). The clinical course of OS makes it a good model for immunotherapy in that even with surgical resection of the primary tumour death occurs in 80% of cases (due to lung metastases within 24 months of resection of the primary tumour) within 30 months. Radiotherapy or single agent chemotherapy does not increase survival rate. Our group (Levin *et al.*, 1975; Byers *et al.*, 1979) investigated the immunoprophylactic potency of OS specific dialyzable leukocyte extract (DLE) (*vide infra*) against lung metastases in humans; the results were promising as five out of six patients without previous overt tumours who received the material for 24 months survived for at least five years.

We have developed an experimental model for evaluating the effect of various immunomodulators on human tumour grown in hamsters previously selectively tolerized to the tumour *in utero*. Injection of tumour specific antigen derived from human OS cells into the foetus *in utero* tolerized the animals. Subsequent injection of live human OS into hamsters produces OS-specific dialysable leukocyte extracts (DLE) and this can be used as a model to evaluate OS-specific DLE; this agent

THEORIES AND MODELS
IN CELLULAR TRANSFORMATION

given after surgical removal of the tumour at 15 days, dramatically increased the survival time (60% survival, 330 days),
whereas DLE devoid of this specificity produced no increase in
survival time. In animals given saline instead of DLE, 60%
survival time was 30 days, (100% mortality by 90 days).

   The incidence of microscopic pulmonary metastases was also
dramatically decreased at 60 days by DLE-OSAA (20% metastases,
control 100%). In contrast, without prior resection of the
primary OS, the DLE-OSAA, even if given immediately after the
tumours were palpable, had no significant prophylactic effect
on pulmonary metastases or on survival.

   Thus, this model gives results closely similar if not identical to that of human osteosarcoma in that DLE OSAA-specific
but not other DLE often prevents death from metastases, but
only if the primary tumour has first been removed.

METHODS

Implantation of Human Osteosarcoma in Hamsters

Inbred LSH/SsLAK hamsters were used. In brief, laparotomy
was performed on pregnant (12 days of gestation) hamsters,
uterus exposed, and the foetuses (6-8 per hamster)
identified. Osteosarcoma associated antigens partially
purified from 2×10^6 TE-85 cells (Singh *et al.* 1976)
(OS human cell line) (100 μg) in 0.1 ml of medium 199 were
injected into each foetus through the intact uterine wall.
After birth, 2×10^6 cells (TE-85-M-MSV) (Singh *et al.*, 1979)
suspended in 0.2 ml of medium 199 were injected adjacent to
the midshaft of the foetus of four-day-old newborn hamsters
(previously injected with osteosarcoma associated antigens in
the foetal stage).

Production of DLE Containing TF for Osteosarcoma Associated Antigens (OSAA)

The method described by us (Singh *et al.*, 1976) was used for
the extraction of plasma membrane and purification of plasma
membrane associated OSAA from TE-85 cells. 500 μg of OSAA
were used for immunization of rabbits. OSAA was injected
intradermally into all four extremities of a female New Zea-
land White rabbit (9-10 lbs) at weekly intervals for three
consecutive weeks. Control groups were injected with (a) PPD
0.85% NaCl and (b) other tumour antigens. For PPD injections
200 mg of PPD were used for the first and second weeks. Two
ml of complete Freund's adjuvant were used for the third week.

Preparation of DLE

Each type of DLE was prepared from peripheral blood leukocytes
by the method of Levin *et al.* (1975), three weeks after antigen
injection. (a) OS specific DLE (DLE-OSAA) was prepared from
rabbits immunized with OSAA. Skin testing was performed on
immunized rabbits. Only those rabbits that showed strong
positive skin tests were used as donors for DLE preparation.
(b) DLE prepared from PPD immunized rabbits (DLE-PPD). (c)
DLE prepared from 0.85% NaCl injected rabbits (DLE-NaCl)
(Fig. 1). The specificity of each DLE preparation was assayed
by LAI and skin test against various antigen preparations and
the results are shown in Fig. 2.

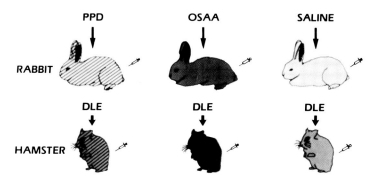

FIG. 1 *Various antigens used for DLE preparation*

Treatment of OS-Bearing Hamsters

Beginning at one day after amputation DLE was administered
subcutaneously into OS-bearing hamsters twice per week for
the first six months and then twice monthly; each injection
contained DLE derived from 10^7 rabbit leukocytes.

For each experiment tumour-bearing hamsters were amputated
when the tumour was palpable in order to remove the tumour
mass. The animals were divided into four groups of ten animals each. Group 1 was treated by amputation alone; group 2,
by amputation plus DLE-OSAA; group 3, by amputation plus DLE-
PPD; group 4, by amputation plus DLE-NaCl.

Assays for Cell Mediated Immunity

In vitro cell-mediated immunity of the DLE treated hamsters
was evaluated by both leukocyte adherence inhibition (LAI)
(Burger *et al.*, 1977) and lymphocyte DNA synthesis (LDS)
(Adkinson *et al.*, 1974). For the LDS assay, lymphocytes were
used at 0.5×10^5 cells/well. One μCi of [^{3}H]-leucine was

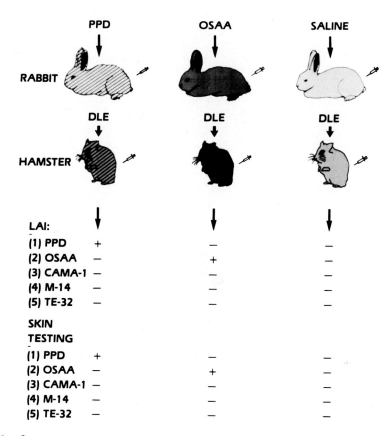

FIG. 2 *Specificity of various DLE preparations*

added to each culture. OSAA was used in a concentration of
20 µg/well. KCl extracts of CAMA-1 cell (breast cancer cell
line) were used as control. After 4 h the cultures were har-
vested. The results, expressed as stimulation index (SI),
were obtained by dividing the average counts per minute with
antigen by the average count per minute of control culture
without antigen. Ear swelling assays at 24 h were also used
as a measure of delayed cutaneous hypersensitivity.

RESULTS

Animal Model

Tumours became palpable 10-15 days following cell inoculation
(Fig. 3). The longest survival was 49 days after tumour
development and the mean survival time was 36 days. Light

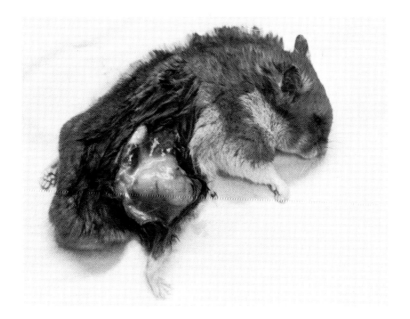

FIG. 3 *Hamster with human sarcoma*

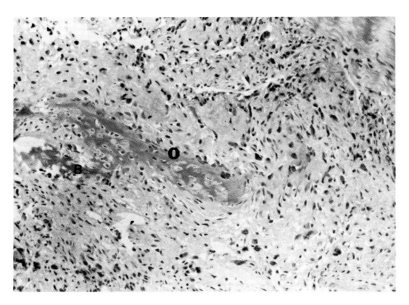

FIG. 4 *Photomicrograph of undecalcified section of a tumour developing adjacent to the femur showing new bone (B) and osteoid (O) formation (X 360).*

TABLE 1

Effects of various preparations of DLE on tumour metastasis

Treatment	Months after amputation										
	0.5	1	2	3	4	5	6	7	8	9	10
Group 1 No DLE	0/10 (0)	6/10 (60)	10/10 (100)								
Group 2 DLE-OSAA	0/10 (0)	0/10 (0)	2/10 (20)	2/10 (20)	3/10 (30)	4/10 (40)	5/10 (50)	5/10 (50)	6/10 (60)	6/10 (60)	6/10 (60)
Group 3 DLE-PPD	0/10 (0)	5/10 (50)	10/10 (100)								
Group 4 DLE-NaCl	0/10 (0)	4/10 (40)	10/10 (100)								

Ten animals were used in each treatment group

Results are expressed in $\dfrac{\text{Number of animals developing metastases}}{\text{Total number of animals}}$

Parentheses = % of animals which developed metastases

microscopy study of the induced tumours indicated that they
were invasive and destructive of the host bone and muscle
tissue. New bone and osteoid were present in variable amounts
(Fig. 4). Light microscopy of the pulmonary tissue showed an
extremely cellular field containing pleomorphic cells with
hyperchromatic nuclei. The malignant cells were invading and
replacing normal pulmonary tissue (Fig. 5). Examination of
92 cells from the induced tumour in the third passage of tissue
culture indicated that the cells had the chromosomal characteristics and the marker chromosome of the cultured TE-85 cells
(Fig. 6).

Effects of DLE on Tumour Metastasis

Table 1 shows the incidence of the pulomnary metastases in
amputated OS bearing hamsters after treatment with different
types of DLE. No mestastasis was seen in any of the four groups
at 0.5 months after amputation. All the animals in any of the
control groups (1,3 and 4) developed pulmonary metastases
within 2 months post amputation. In contrast, only 2 of the
10 animals in group 2 developed metastases within 2 months
post amputation. (At 10 months post amputation, of the 10
animals in this group, 6 had pulmonary metastases.)

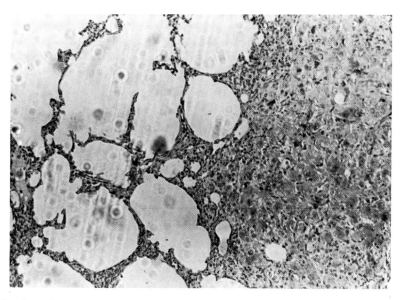

FIG. 5 *Photomicrography of section of the pulmonary tissue
showing malignant cells in the right and normal lung tissue
of the left (X 240)*

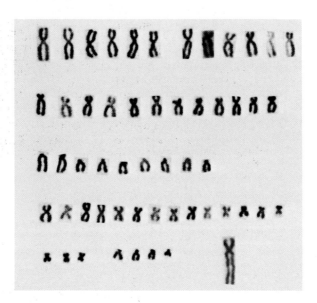

FIG. 6 *Karyotype of hamster induced tumour cells.   Chromosome number is 55.   A marker chromosome with submedian centromer is seen in the bottom row*

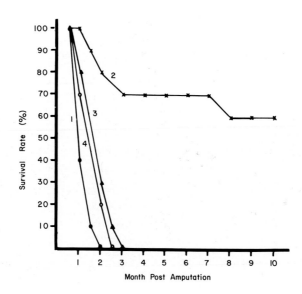

FIG. 7 *Effect of DLE on the survival time of OS-hamsters.* ● – *amputation alone (group 1);* **X** – *treated with DLE-OSAA (group 2);* ▲ – *treated with DLE-PPD (group 3);* O – *treated with DLE-NaCl (group 4).*

Effects of DLE on the Survival Time

The survival rate of OS-hamsters receiving treatment with
various types of DLE are shown in Fig. 7. Sixty per cent of
the DLE-OSAA treated animals were still alive at 330 days post
amputation. (All animals in groups 1,3 and 4 died within
one to three months post amputation.)

Effects of DLE on Cell Mediated Immunity

Figures 8 and 9 show the results of the LAI reactivity on the
animals treated with various types of DLE at 0.5 month and 1
month post amputation. Adherence inhibition of less than 20%
was not significantly different from controls as previously
determined in our laboratory. Animals in groups 1,3 and 4
had low LAI reactivities at 0.5 month and 1 month post amputation. Only 2 of the 10 animals in group 2 had decreased LAI
reactivity at 1 month post amputation. Figure 10 shows the
results of LAI reactivity at 0.5 month post amputation when a
KCl extract of CAMA-1 cells was used as antigen source. The
LAI reactivity was at the control level in all four groups.
The results of the lymphocyte DNA synthesis activity at 0.5
month and 1 month post amputation are shown in Figs. 11 and 12.
The SI in groups 1,3 and 4 animals were low when determined
at 0.5 month and 1 month post amputation. Only 2 of the 10

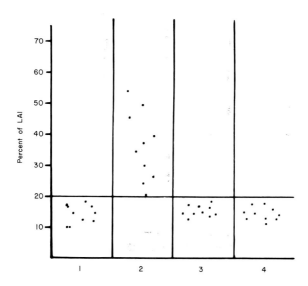

FIG. 8 *Effect of DLE on LAI activity of OS-hamsters at 0.5
month post amputation. (1) Amputation alone; (2) treated with
DLE-OSAA; (3) treated with DLE-PPD; (4) treated with DLE-NaCl.*

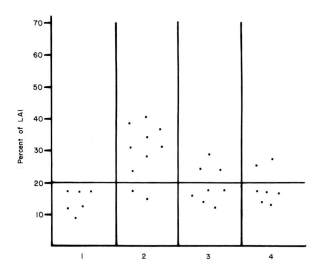

FIG. 9 *Effect of DLE on LAI activity of OS-hamsters at 1 month post amputation. (1) Amputation alone; (2) treated with DLE-OSAA; (3) treated with DLE-PPD; (4) treated with DLE-NaCl.*

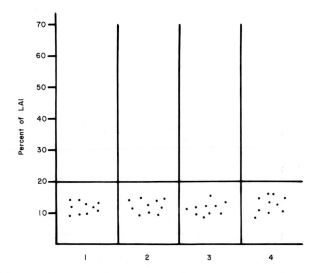

FIG. 10 *LAI activity of OS-hamsters at 0.5 month post amputation with KCl extract from CAMA-1 cells used as antigen source.*

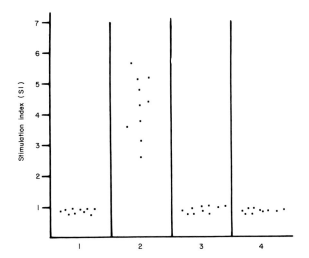

FIG. 11 *Effect of DLE on lymphocyte DNA synthesis of OS-
hamsters at 0.5 month post amputation. (1) Amputation alone;
(2) DLE-OSAA; (3) DLE-PPD; (4) DLE-NaCl. Results are expressed
in stimulation index (SI) (see Materials and Methods)*

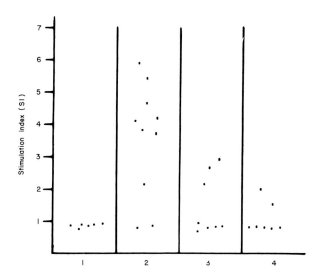

FIG. 12 *Effect of DLE on lymphocyte DNA synthesis of OS-
hamsters at 1 month post amputation. (1) Amputation alone;
(2) DLE-OSAA; (3) DLE-PPD; (4) DLE-NaCl. Results are expressed
in stimulation index (SI) (see Materials and Methods)*

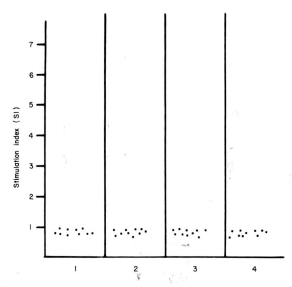

FIG. 13 *Lymphocyte DNA synthesis activity of OS hamsters at 0.5 month post amputation with KCl extracts of CAMA-1 cells used as antigen source. (1) Amputation alone; (2) DLE-OSAA; (3) DLE-PPD; (4) DLE-NaCl. Results are expressed in stimulation index (SI) (see Materials and Methods)*

animals in group 2 had decreased LDS at 1 month post amputation. As shown in Fig. 13, when a KCl extract of CAMA-1 cells was used as antigen source, the results of LDS activity was at the control level in all animals. Tables 2 and 3 show the results of LAI activity and LDS activity of the surviving animals in group 2 at 4 and 8 months post amputation. Both LAI reactivity and LDS were significantly higher ($p < 0.001$) with OSAA antigen than with KCl extracts of CAMA-1 cells as antigen source.

DISCUSSION

In the present investigation, we attempted to extend the life-span of hamsters by amputation removal of the primary tumour mass. We used OS-specific DLE for prophylaxis against pulmonary metastases, the cause of rapid death in such animals bearing human OS. The survival rate in the DLE-OSAA group in a 330 day period was much higher (60%) in the DLE-OSAA treated group as compared to the control groups which comprised amputation alone, DLE-PPD treated and DLE-NaCl treated (all are 0%). The rate of pulmonary metastases in a 300 day period is lower in the DLE-OSAA treated group (60%) as compared to the control groups (100%). It should be emphasized that the DLE

TABLE 2

*Effect of DLE-OSAA on the cell-mediated immunity
of the surviving animal at 4 months post amputation*

Animal number	LAI[a]		SI[b]	
	OSAA	CAMA-1	OSAA	CAMA-1
1	50.1±8.6*	15.1±2.3	7.23±0.4*	1.09±0.2
2	44.2±7.5*	10.2±1.4	5.06±0.8*	0.92±0.1
3	40.1±6.3*	10.4±1.9	4.01±0.3*	1.03±0.09
4	41.4±7.2*	11.4±1.2	6.14±0.2*	0.98±0.07
5	53.4±9.1*	12.0±0.8	7.62±1.6*	0.89±0.1
6	46.2±7.3*	10.5±1.7	4.31±1.8*	1.06±0.3
7	37.4±6.1*	16.4±0.6	4.02±0.9*	0.97±0.2

20 µg of antigens were used in both assays

*Significant. $p < 0.001$ as determined by Student's t test

OSAA = osteosarcoma associated antigens

CAMA-1 = KCl extracts of CAMA-1 cells

[a]Results are expressed in % of leukocyte adherence inhibition

[b]SI = stimulation index ($\frac{\text{cpm with antigen}}{\text{cpm without antigen}}$)

was derived from a different species (rabbit) than the recipient. One of us (Klesius *et al.*, 1978; Klesius *et al.*, 1979) previously reported the interspecies transfer of cell mediated immunity (CMI) from cattle to mice. CMI to *Eimeria ferrisi* was stimulated in mice by treatment with bovine DLE prepared from cattle immune to *Eimeria bovis*. The DLE derived from cattle immune to clinical coccidiosis stimulated lymphocytes in the hosts to preserve function in a protective CMI response. We therefore decided to use rabbit DLE in this study because of easy access to animals of this species. Our group (Levin *et al.*, 1975; Byers *et al.*, 1979) previously reported the clinical and immunological parameters in osteosarcoma patients given DLE. Of 7 patients with primary tumours not removed at the beginning of OS specific DLE therapy, there was no increase in survival time as compared with historical controls (Marcove *et al.*, 1971). However, 5 of the 6 patients following

TABLE 3

*Effect of DLE-OSAA on the cell-mediated immunity
of the surviving animal at 8 months post amputation*

Animal number	LAI[a]		SI[b]	
	OSAA	CAMA-1	OSAA	CAMA-1
1	41.2±4.5*	11.4±0.8	5.10±0.1*	0.96±0.2
2	40.0±6.9*	9.2±0.4	4.34±0.5*	0.81±0.1
3	ND	ND	ND	0.85±0.1
4	35.1±5.6*	8.4±0.3	3.26±0.3*	1.05±0.2
5	32.4±0.3*	11.6±0.8	4.67±0.1*	0.82±0.4
6	34.6±5.4*	10.9±0.7	3.12±0.2*	0.94±0.2
7	42.4±8.7*	12.4±1.0	2.36±0.4*	1.02±0.6

[a]Results are expressed in % of leukocyte adherence inhibition

[b]SI = stimulation index $(\frac{\text{cpm with antigen}}{\text{cpm without antigen}})$

20 μg of antigens were used in both assays

*Significant, $p < 0.001$ as determined by Student's t test

OSAA = osteosarcoma associated antigens

CAMA-1 = KCl extracts of CAMA-1 cells

ND = not done

tumour resection apparently free of overt metastases at the
initiation of OS-specific DLE therapy were alive and disease
free at last follow-up, 62-82 months after surgery. Compared
with the probabilities of five years survival computed from
historical controls, this is highly significant ($p < 0.008$).
This increase in survival time due to prevention of pulmonary
metastases in patients treated with OS specific DLE is in con-
cordance with the animal model. In this study the CMI as
measured by LAI and LDS were strikingly low in animal and control groups 1,3 and 4 at 0.5 month post amputation. (This
phenomenon may be due to the removal of the primary tumour
from the host; decrease of tumour specific CMI in the host
after tumour removal has been reported by other investigators
(Levin *et al.*, 1975; Camblin *et al.*, 1977; Fisher *et al.*,
1976). Both LAI and LDS activity in experimental animals

were high when measured at 0.5 month, 1 month, 4 months, and 8 months; suggesting that administration of DLE-OSAA increased OS specific CMI. Three of the animals in group 3, and two of the animals in group 4 had increased LAI and LDS activity when measured at 1 month. This result may be due to the presence of micrometastases but not widespread metastases in the host. The low LAI and LDS activity in most of the animals in the control groups at 1 month presumably is due to the presence of tumour metastases in these animals. These results are similar to our findings (Levin *et al.*, 1975) that CMI of OS patients increased dramatically after injection of OS-tumour specific DLE. The results reported in this investigation indicate that OS-hamsters given DLE-OSAA after amputation have a better survival rate, far exceeding animals treated by (a) amputation alone, or (b) DLE-PPD lacking OS specific transfer factor or (c) DLE-NaCl. The evidence of the capability of DLE-OSAA to enhance specific CMI against OS is reflected by the increases in LAI and LDS activity.

DLE immunotherapy has been used for treatment of various types of tumours. The animal model described here is unique, and the DLE-OSAA is specific and can be used for further investigation of the other effects of osteosarcoma specific DLE alone and in combination with other immunomodulating and chemotherapeutic agents in the therapy of human osteosarcoma. The information obtained from these studies appears relevant to the treatment of osteosarcoma in humans. In addition, this animal model can be used in the evaluation of the effectiveness of various immune potentiating drugs; and be individualized to a given point. We have had success for results with new chemotherapeutic agents in this model.

Regarding the ability of the transfer moiety in DLE to increase tumour specific cytotoxicity, we believe that it may be occurring through a TF-mediated release of cytotoxic precursor lymphocytes (CTL-P) from a set of CTL-P cells as well as clonal expansion of specific precursor lymphocytes.

Dialysable transfer factor was first reported in 1955 by Lawrence (1955); he reported that dialysable leukocyte extracts (DLE) from donors with positive skin rest reactions to PPD could transfer skin test positivity when injected into recipients who previously were skin test negative. Our group (Levin *et al.*, 1980) subsequently demonstrated that DLE could also transfer the ability to produce chemical mediators of cell mediated immunity (CMI), such as macrophage migration inhibitory factor (MIF). DLE also causes a rise in the level of active rosette-forming cells (Wybran *et al.*, 1973), a T-cell subset which appears to measure the sum total of the efferent limb of cell-mediated immunity in recipients with deficient CMI (Fudenberg *et al.*, 1976). DLE has since been used both

therapeutically and prophylactically in patients with one or
another genetically determined deficiency in CMI (Levin *et al.*,
1970) as well as in a variety of other diseases (Spitler *et
al.*, 1972; Arala-Chaves *et al.*, 1978; Fudenberg *et al.*, 1976).
Only one of the 200 components in DLE transfers antigen specific reactivity. This one is termed transfer factor. Recently,
a randomized, double-blind, placebo-controlled trial was conducted in a large group of children with acute leukaemia in
remission, a group known to have high susceptibility to varicella zoster encephalitis; using DLEs from five donors with
unusually high *in vitro* reactivity to varicella zoster antigens, long term prophylaxis against varicella was achieved
after a single DLE injection (Steele, 1980); DLEs from donors
devoid of such activity to varicella had no prophylactic
effect. We have subsequently used DLE in a tumour model in
an attempt to delineate its mechanism.

The success of DLE in clinical trials in humans reported
to date has been inconsistent, even for a single disease or
syndrome; but this is hardly surprising in view of the heterogeneity of DLE preparations and, especially, of the many different methods used (or not used at all) for selecting donors
and monitoring the progress of recipients. On one point, however, there is almost univeral agreement: DLE has remarkably
few side effects and is perhaps the safest immunotherapeutic
modality now in clinical use (Arala-Chaves *et al.*, 1978).

The importance of immunologic assays for the clinical use
of DLE (containing TF) cannot be overemphasized. Indeed, we
believe that much of the current controversy regarding the
efficacy of DLE in the treatment of various immunodeficiencies,
malignancies, and infections (viral, mycobacterial, and para-
sitic) diseases can be attributed to (a) failure to select
suitable donors and (b) failure to individualize the therapeutic regimen for each recipient. The importance of donor
selection lies in the apparent antigen-specific nature of the
TF component(s) in DLE. If, for example, a patient with
disseminated candidiasis refractory to antifungal agents (perhaps due to an antigen-selective defect of cellular immunity)
is to be treated, it is obvious that the leukocyte donor(s)
should be selected on the basis of demonstrable strong cell-
mediated immunity (CMI) to *Candida* antigen. This situation
is complicated, however, by the fact that DLE preparations
contain (in addition to the antigen-specific TF moieties) non-
specific adjuvant activities and in some preparations one or
more inhibitory activities (Wilson and Fudenberg, 1979; Wilson
et al., 1979a and b; Wilson *et al.*, 1980; Wilson *et al.*,
1983b). Thus, some clinical improvement may be seen in
patients receiving DLE of the "wrong" antigenic specificity,
due to the adjuvant effect; and DLE of the "right" specificity

may be ineffective if the preparation lacks potency or contains excess amounts of inhibitory material. Complete purification and chemical synthesis of the antigen-specific TF activity will be of enormous benefit in resolving the preceding problems (our progress towards these goals is discussed later in this review). Until this is accomplished, however, the best approach to DLE immunotherapy and/or immunoprophylaxis is the use of standard-ized immunologic assays for careful selection of donors, test-ing for specificity and potency of TF in DLE preparations *in vitro* before administration, and monitoring of recipients so that DLE will be used in sufficient quantity and with appro-priate frequency (Fudenberg *et al.*, 1983; Wilson *et al.*, 1982). Different patients may exhibit varying responses to the immuno-modulating effects of the same batch of DLE (so-called "recip-ient specificity") (Arala-Chaves and Fudenberg, 1976; Arala-Chaves *et al.*, 1977). Moreover, the immune system of each patient can be regarded as a "teeter-totter" balancing immune competence against antigen load: when the antigenic burden exceeds the protective capacity of the immune system the dis-ease progresses; when the situation is reversed, clinical im-provement follows. Thus, the immune competence of each DLE recipient must be monitored regularly by appropriate immuno-logical tests, so that additional DLE can be administered when the balance begins to shift. This requirement for individual-ized therapy is analogous to the clinical management of insulin-dependent diabetics, where for each patient the amount and frequency of insulin administration must be determined on the basis of the individual's particular clinical status, and variations occur in a single individual as a result of infec-tion or changes in diet, exercise habits, or other factors.

In addition to transfer factor, DLE contains many other moieties with biological activity. DLE can inhibit the spon-taneous resynthesis of shed Fc receptors by normal leukocytes (Nekam *et al.*, 1978), shows a marked increase in ADCC in patients with low ADCC before DLE therapy (Nekam *et al.*, 1978), and causes significant stimulation of natural killer (NK) cell activity both *in vivo* and *in vitro* in patients with low cyto-toxicity capacity before therapy (Lang *et al.*, 1982); and has adjuvant moieties as well. These effects may be operative in our OS-DLE model discussed herein, but seem precluded by lack of effect immunologically or clinically of DLEs lacking OSAA-TF. In terms of structure, TF appears to be an RNA peptide of about 2530 MW. Our present data suggest that TF-H5 has internal purine residues and a peptide at the N-terminal (Wilson *et al.*, 1979c, 1981, 1983a).

We have also examined bovine TF specific for PPD (Wilson *et al.*, 1982). The bovine TF, unlike human TF, was prepared by an "incubation release method" (Klesius and Fudenberg,

1977) and is structurally similar to TF-H5 except that it lacks a 2' or 3'-terminal phosphate (Wilson *et al.*, 1982). Presumably the human counterpart is present in material extracted from human T cells *in vivo*.

Immunologists seeing the above data concerning putative structure and biologic activity of transfer factor for the first time invariably ask how such a small molecule can really work in a specific manner and how can such a small molecule have so many different effects and account for so many specificities? The data suggest that a given transfer factor contains perhaps eight or nine bases and six to eight amino acids. Presumably, we all have a million or more different "transfer factors", and an immunologically virgin cell, when encountering transfer factor of one specificity, binds this TF to the cell surface, whereas a second already committed cell would not bind TF of a second specificity. Presumably a second TF of a different specificity binds to a second virgin cell and a third immunocyte binds yet another different transfer factor within the same DLE preparation. Thus, the penultimate query might reside in which (and when) particular immunocytes possess receptors for TF. Since 6 amino acids are compatible with the size of the third hypervariable region in immunoglobulins, if we assume that any of the 20 known amino acids can occupy any of the 6 positions the number of possible combinations, each conferring a different immunologic specificity, can provide more than 6.4×10^6 differing specificities. Most immunologists estimate the number of different specificities present in each individual as somewhere between 10,000 (Talmadge, 1959) and 10 million. Hence with 6 amino acids each individual could have more than 6 million TFs; enough to account for all antigenic encounters. The hypothesis that a structure with 6 amino acids serves as antigen receptor is especially intriguing to us in view of the reports by Kabat that the antigen binding site of antibody molecules (at least for various dextrans) encompasses about 6 residues (Kabat, 1966). Again further experiments are warranted. It appears not unlikely that TF of a given specificity may be the T cell antigen receptor (or a portion thereof) for epitopes of that specificity.

SUMMARY

An experimental model for evaluating the effect of immunomodulators on human tumour grown in hamsters previously selectively tolerized to the tumour *in utero* has been developed. We show that human osteosarcoma (OS) can be grown *in vivo* after injection of live OS cells into newborn hamsters previously tolerized *in utero* with semi-purified OS antigen; this model can be used to evaluate tumour-specific immunomodulation. OS-specific dialysable leukocyte extracts (DLE), for example, given after surgical removal of the tumour at 15 days, dramatically increased the survival time (60% survival, 300 days), whereas DLE with other specificity or devoid of known specificity produced no increase in survival time. (Dialysable leukocyte extracts (DLE) has been used both therapeutically and prophylactically in patients with genetically determined deficiency in CMI as well as in a variety of other diseases. The antigen-specific transfer factor in DLE responsible for improvement is an RNA-peptide MW about 2500).

The incidence of microscopic pulmonary metastases was also dramatically decreased at 60 days by DLE-OSAA (20% metastases, control 100%), but not by DLE with other specificities, e.g. DLE-PPD. Without prior resection of the primary OS, the DLE-OSAA, even if given immediately after the tumours were palpable, had no significant prophylactic effect on metastases. Thus, this "model" behaves biologically in a manner closely similar if not identical to that of humans with osteosarcoma in that DLE-OSAA but not other DLE often prevents death from pulmonary metastases, but only if the primary tumour has first been removed (Fudenberg et al., Perspect. Virol. IX, 1975).

We have used this model to test the immunomodulating effects of several classes of drugs, e.g. isoprinosine and NPT-15392 which reverse immunosuppression, and IAHQ, a new 2-amino-4-hydroxyquinazalone that inhibits the enzyme thymidylate synthase and appears to selectively kill or inactivate suppressor (as opposed to helper) T cells; the sum total of data suggests that the decrease in pulmonary metastases and thus enhanced life is due to inactivation of suppressor T cells by either the drugs or as a sequela of OS-DLE administration. Hence the model lends itself to studies of abolition of "tolerance" (decrease in antigen-specific suppressor T cells) in the foetus and the neonate and the immunological differentiation of suppressor T cells into cytotoxic T cells. Preliminary data, in contrast to current dogma, suggest that the same cell (Leu 2^+) thought to have both antigen-specific cytotoxic function for OS cells and antigen-specific "suppressor" function, are in reality separate populations. How DLE-TF (and/or other components within DLE) cause a switch from active suppressor to cytotoxic cells is currently under study; perhaps it is by differential effects on CTL precursors.

ACKNOWLEDGEMENTS

Publication no. 632 from the Department of Basic and Clinical Immunology and Microbiology, Medical University of South Carolina. Research supported in part by USPHS Grant CA-25746.

REFERENCES

Adkinson, N.F., Rosenberg, S.A. and Terry, W.D. (1974). *J. Immunol.* 112, 1426.

Arala-Chaves, M.P. and Fudenberg, H.H. (1976). *Nature* 263, 155-156.

Arala-Chaves, M.P., Silva, A., Porto, M.T., Picoto, A., Ramos, M.T.F. and Fudenberg, H.H. (1977). *Clin. Immunol. Immunopathol.* 8, 430-447.

Arala-Chaves, M.P., Hormanheimo, M., Goust, J.M. and Fudenberg, H.H. (1978). *In* "Immunological Engineering" (Ed. D.W. Jirsch), pp.35-82. MTP Press Ltd., London.

Arala-Chaves, M.P., Klesius, P.H. and Fudenberg, H.H. (1979). *In* "Immune Regulators in Transfer Factor" (Eds. A. Khan, C.H. Kirkpatrick and N.O. Hills), pp.15-25. Academic Press, New York.

Burger, D.R., Vandenbark, A.A., Finke, P., Malley, A., Frikke, M., Black, J., Acott, K., Begley, D. and Vetto, R.M. (1977). *J. Natl. Cancer Inst.* 59, 317-324.

Byers, V.S., LeCam, L., Levin, A.S., Johnston, J.O. and Hackett, A.J. (1979). *Cancer Immunol. Immunother.* 6, 243-253.

Camblin, J., Enneking, W., Forbes, J. and Smith, R. (1977). *In* "Neoplasm Immunity" (Ed. R.G. Crispen), pp.201-210. Inst. Press, Philadelphia.

Cortes, E.P., Holland, J.F. and Glidewell, O. (1978). *Cancer Treat. Rep.* 62, 271-277.

Dahlin, D.C. and Coventry, M.B. (1967). *J. Bone Joint Surg.* 49, 101-110.

Fisher, B., Wolmark, N., Coyle, J. and Saffer, E.A. (1976). *Cancer Res.* 36, 2302-2305.

Fudenberg, H.H., Goust, J.M., Arala-Chaves, M.P. and Wilson, G.B. (1976). *Folia, Allerg. Immunol.* 23, 1-23.

Fudenberg, H.H., Wilson, G.B., Keller, R.H., Metcalf, J.F., Paulling, E.E., Stuart, E.J. and Floyd, E. (1983). *In* "Fourth International Transfer Factor Workshop" (Eds. C.H. Kirkpatrick, H.S. Lawrence and D.R. Burger). Academic Press, in press.

Jaffe, N., Frei, G., Watts, H. and Traggis, D. (1978). *Cancer Treat. Rep.* 62, 259-264.

Kabat, E.A. (1966). *J. Immunol.* 97, 1.

Klesius, P. and Fudenberg, H.H. (1977). *Clin. Immunol. Immunopathol.* 8, 238-246.

Klesius, P.H., Qualls, D.F., Elston, A.L. and Fudenberg, H.H. (1978). *Clin. Immunol. Immunopathol.* 10, 214-221.

Klesius, P.H., Elston, A.L., Chambers, W.H. and Fudenberg, H.H. (1979). *Clin. Immunol. Immunopathol.* 12, 143-149.

Lang, I., Nekam, K., Gergeley, P. and Petranyi, Gy. (1982).

Clin. Immunol. Immunopathol. 25, 139.

Lawrence, H.S. (1955). *J. Clin. Invest.* 34, 219-230.

Levin, A.S., Spitler, L.E., Stites, D.P. and Fudenberg, H.H. (1970). *Proc. Natl. Acad. Sci. USA* 67, 821-828.

Levin, A.S., Byers, V.S., Fudenberg, H.H., Wybran, J., Hackett, A.J., Johnston, J.O. and Spitler, L.E. (1975). *J. Clin. Invest.* 55, 487-499.

Marcove, R.C., Mike, V., Hajek, J.V., Levin, A.G. and Hutter, R.V.P. (1971). *NY State J. Med.* 71, 855-866.

Nekam, K., Lang, I., Fekete, B., Gergely, P. and Petranyi, Gy. (1978). *Acta Microbiol. Acad. Sci. Hung.* 25, 191.

Singh, I., Tsang, K.Y. and Blakemore, W.S. (1976). *Cancer Res.* 36, 4130-4136.

Singh, I., Tsang, K.Y. and Blakemore, W.S. (1979). *Clin. Orthop. Rel. Res.* 144, 305-310.

Spitler, L.E., Levin, A.S., Stites, D.P., Fudenberg, H.H., Pirofsky, B., August, C.S., Stiehm, E.R., Hitzig, W.H. and Gatti, R.A. (1972). *J. Clin. Invest.* 51, 3216-3224.

Steele, R.W. (1980). *Cell Immunol.* 50, 282-289.

Sutow, W.W., Gehan, F.A., Vietto, T.J., Frias, A.E. and Dyment, P.G. (1976). *J. Bone Joint Surg.* 58A, 629-633 (Abstract).

Talmadge, D.W. (1959). *Science* 129, 1643.

Wilson, G.B. and Fudenberg, H.H. (1979). *J. Lab. Clin. Med.* 93, 819-837.

Wilson, G.B., Fudenberg, H.H. and Horsmanheimo, M. (1979a). *J. Lab. Clin. Med.* 93, 800-818.

Wilson, G.B., Smith, C.L. and Fudenberg, H.H. (1979b). *J. Allergy Clin. Immunol.* 64, 56-66.

Wilson, G.B., Paddock, G.V. and Fudenberg, H.H. (1979c). *Trans. Soc. Amer. Phys.* 92, 239-256.

Wilson, G.B., Fudenberg, H.H., Jonnson, H.T. Jr. and Smith, C.L. (1980). *Clin. Immunol. Immunopathol.* 16, 90-112.

Wilson, G.B., Paddock, G.V. and Fudenberg, H.H. (1981). *Thymus* 2, 257-276.

Wilson, G.B., Paddock, G.V. and Fudenberg, H.H. (1982). *Thymus* 4, 335-350.

Wilson, G.B., Metcalf, J.F. Jr. and Fudenberg, H.H. (1982). *Clin. Immunol. Immunopathol.* 23, 478-491.

Wilson, G.B., Paddock, G.V., Floyd, E., Newell, R.T. and Dopson, M.H. (1983a). *In* "Immunobiology of Transfer Factor" (Eds. C.H. Kirkpatrick, H.S. Lawrence and D.R. Burger), pp.395-410. Academic Press, New York.

Wilson, G.B., Paddock, G.V., Floyd, E., Newell, R.T. and Dopson, M.H. (1983b). *In* "Fourth International Transfer Factor Workshop" (Eds. C.H. Kirkpatrick, H.S. Lawrence and D.R. Burger), Academic Press, in press.

Wybran, J., Levin, A.S., Spitler, L.E. and Fudenberg, H.H. (1973). *N. Engl. J. Med.* 288, 710-713.

NORMAL AND ABNORMAL MODES OF EXPRESSION OF DEVELOPMENTALLY REGULATED GENES

B. Mintz

The Institute for Cancer Research, Fox Chase Cancer Center, Philadelphia, Pennsylvania, USA

INTRODUCTION

The neoplastic state may be viewed as a developmental aberration (Pierce, 1967; Markert, 1968; Mintz, 1978a,b; Mintz and Fleischman, 1981). According to this view, the target is a stem cell, either relatively early and still multipotential, or more restricted in its fate and unipotential. The impairment is a reduction or loss of the capacity to differentiate. Retention of its proliferative ability can then lead to increasing selection for more rapidly growing variant stem cells, especially in the more malignant or anaplastic tumours. Thus, the problem is basically one of the developmental regulation of gene expression, in many ways the same problem with which we are confronted in attempting to understand the normal development of a complex multicellular organism from the single-celled fertilized egg. In the case of malignancy, the inciting cause may be a mutational change, an oncogenic virus, a hormonal shift, etc. Any one of a number of genes may be the culprit but, in all cases, a regulatory change in gene expression is involved. We will therefore be considering here, first, an experimental study dealing with the relation between malignancy and differentiation; and, next, experiments describing new approaches to the analysis of gene expression during development *in vivo*.

FROM ABNORMAL TO NORMAL GENE EXPRESSION IN MOUSE TERATO-CARCINOMA CELLS

The most striking example of the effect of aberrant gene function on stem cells has been documented in mouse teratocarcinoma

THEORIES AND MODELS
IN CELLULAR TRANSFORMATION

cells. Here, the experimental reversal of the cells from malignancy to normalcy has been achieved by shifting the pattern of gene activity from the proliferative mode into the pathway of differentiation *in vivo*.

Mouse teratocarcinoma stem cells are apparently the malignant counterparts of normal early somatic embryo cells (Mintz, 1978a; Mintz *et al.*, 1978) whose proliferation has been sustained while their differentiation has become limited and chaotic. Various tissues are found in the solid tumours formed when the cells are grown subcutaneously in a syngeneic host; however, these tissues are usually immature and there are many types that are never represented (Stevens, 1967). Derivation of the differentiated cells from the primitive stem cells was demonstrated by the range of cell types obtained after single cells were transplanted to adult recipients (Kleinsmith and Pierce, 1964). The stem cells are capable of being propagated as transplant lines *in vivo* (either in the solid or modified-ascites form) and also as cell culture lines.

If the stem cells were in fact the neoplastic derivatives of developmentally totipotent embryo cells, it seemed possible that their differentiation might become more normal if they were in the company of the corresponding normal stem cells, i.e. if they were placed in early embryos. Such an experiment would be comparable to the production of allophenic mice - animals with cells of different genotypes, produced by bringing together blastomeres from two different embryos (Mintz, 1965a; Mintz, 1974), except that the teratocarcinoma stem cells would be used instead of one of the normal embryonic contributors.

The experiment was carried out by injecting tumour stem cells from a karyotypically normal *in vivo* transplant line into blastocysts of another strain identifiable by numerous genetic markers. The tumour cells were indeed stably "normalized" by the accompanying embryo cells after almost a decade of serial transplantation in the malignant state (Mintz and Illmensee, 1975; Cronmiller and Mintz, 1978). The neoplastic defect was therefore one of aberrant control of gene expression. Tumour-lineage cells were able to contribute, in the best cases, not only to all somatic tissues (along with embryo-lineage cells) but also to functional germ cells and to progeny in which the tumour-cell genome was perpetuated. Successful but more limited differentiation was obtained in related experiments by others in which other tumour stem cells contributed to formation of one (Brinster, 1974) or of several (Papaioannou *et al.*, 1975) somatic tissues, but not of all somatic tissues and never to germ cells.

TERATOCARCINOMA CELLS AS VEHICLES FOR GENE CHANGES IN MICE

The capacity for normal and complete somatic and germinal differentiation in our experiments formed the basis for a novel
experimental scheme: inasmuch as the stem cells could be
grown in culture, they might serve there as "surrogate eggs"
in which selected genetic changes could be made at will; after
injection of the cells into blastocysts, the change could be
ultimately be represented in the germ line and lead to new
strains of mice of predetermined genotype (Mintz, 1978a; Mintz,
1978b; Mintz, 1979). Large numbers of stem cells could be
subjected to specific selection or screening procedures *in
vitro* and only cells with the gene change of interest would be
injected into blastocysts.

In the case of DNA transformation, the teratocarcinoma
route would have certain advantages over the egg-injection
route: many tumour cells could be treated, and selected or
screened; moreover, selected cell clones could be precharacter-
ized, e.g. to ascertain the chromosomal site of DNA integration
by means of *in situ* hybridization. Among the range of options
that the teratocarcinoma experimental system offers is production of animals with murine mutations which would yield mouse
models of a corresponding human genetic disease. Derivation
of mice with mutations in mitochondrial genes would also be
possible (Mintz, 1979; Watanabe *et al.*, 1978).

An example of a relevant human genetic disease is Lesch-
Nyhan disease, due to a severe deficiency of the enzyme hypox-
anthine phosphoribosyltransferase (HPRT). The human disorder
results from an X-linked recessive defect that is usually
fatal in affected males (Lesch and Nyhan, 1964; Seegmiller
et al., 1967). By first selecting mutagenized mouse teratocarcinoma stem cells of an *in vitro* culture line for resistance to the purine base analogue 6-thioguanine, an HPRT-
deficient cell clone was isolated. When these cells were injected into blastocysts of another strain, mosaic animals were
obtained (Dewey *et al.*, 1977). The tumour-strain cellular
population (distinguishable by an independent strain-specific
isozyme marker) had retained the HPRT defect throughout differentiation. Strong selective pressure against the defective
cells in blood of the mosaic animals provided an interesting
parallel to selection against cells of the defective phenotype
in the blood of human heterozygous female carriers.

The cell line used in this HPRT-mutant experiment, and in
all other teratocarcinoma mutagenesis experiments until
recently, was not karyotypically normal, however. The abnormality in the HPRT-deficient case was a trisomy that would not
be compatible with production of viable germ-line progeny
(Gropp, 1975), although it obviously permitted formation of all

somatic tissues (Dewey *et al.*, 1977).

We have also isolated mutant teratocarcinoma cells deficient in other enzymes, such as adenine phosphoribosyltransferase (Reuser and Mintz, 1979) or thymidine kinase (Pellicer *et al.*, 1980); and have laid some of the groundwork for seeking teratocarcinoma mutants with deficiencies in specific receptor systems, such as the low-density lipoprotein receptor (Goldstein *et al.*, 1979) or the transferrin receptor (Karin and Mintz, 1981).

Transfer of recombinant DNA into teratocarcinoma cells has been accomplished for selectable as well as unselectable genes. In our earlier experiments, mutant teratocarcinoma cells that were stably deficient in thymidine kinase activity (tk^-) were first isolated. They were then used as recipients, after addition of DNA in a calcium phosphate precipitate, and selection in HAT (hypoxanthine/aminopterin/thymidine) medium, to obtain cell clones that had taken up the foreign HSV *tk* gene (Pellicer *et al.*, 1980), as in previous experiments (Wigler *et al.*, 1977; Wigler *et al.*, 1978) carried out with fibroblast cell lines. Cotransfer of the unselectable human β-globin gene, by inclusion in the precipitate along with the HSV *tk* gene, was successful in some tk^+ transformants (Pellicer *et al.*, 1980).

More recently, we have treated tk^- teratocarcinoma stem cells with DNA from the same plasmid vector, PtkHβ1, as was used in this laboratory for DNA injection into the pronucleus of fertilized eggs. The unselectable human β-globin gene was linked to the selectable HSV *tk* gene in the bacterial plasmid. A high transformation efficiency was obtained after selection in HAT (Wagner and Mintz, 1982). Hybridization tests disclosed the presence of intact copies (three to six per cell) of the human gene in the majority of transformants. That these donor sequences were associated with cellular DNA was inferred from the presence of some new high molecular weight fragments, seen in Southern blots, and from stability of the donor sequences in tumours resulting from subcutaneous injection of the cells.

In order to test for production of mRNA transcripts of the human gene, total polyadenylate-containing RNA was examined in four of the transformed cultured cell clones. Two of these showed hybridization to the human-gene probe. The RNA species from one of them resembled mature transcripts of the human β-globin gene; the others were larger in size (Wagner and Mintz, 1982). Erythroid development was seen in some of the tumours, although it is not yet known whether any of the haemoglobin in them was attributable to the foreign gene.

Dominant-selection vectors enable recombinant genetic material to be transferred to wild-type cells, thereby circumventing the initial mutagenesis and selection steps (e.g. to obtain tk^- mutant recipient cells). This could help to avoid

occurrence of extraneous and undesirable genetic changes during
the initial phases of gene transfer into teratocarcinoma cells
in culture. The plasmid DNA vectors (pSV-*gpt*, from P. Berg),
carrying the *E. coli* bacterial gene for xanthine-guanine phosphoribosyltransferase and some regulatory sequences from SV40,
in addition to pBR322 (Mulligan and Berg, 1980; Mulligan and
Berg, 1981), have provided such an opportunity. We have isolated numerous transformants after addition of pSV2-*gpt* DNA in
calcium phosphate to the cell culture medium and selection in
mycophenolic acid (Wagner and Mintz, 1982). The donor DNA
sequences were apparently stably integrated into the stem cells
and their differentiated tumour derivatives. We may conclude
that any cloned gene can now be introduced into teratocarcinoma
stem cells, even without mutagenesis of the cells, by cotransfer with, or linked transfer in, such vectors. New
hybridization methods allowing *in situ* chromosomal visual-
ization of genes (Robins *et al.*, 1981) should make it possible
to precharacterize the transformants and to choose those of
interest for experiments involving further differentiation in
the soma and in the germ line *in vivo*.

A limitation in the teratocarcinoma "portal of entry"
scheme has heretofore been the lack of a cell culture line
characterized by karyotypic normalcy and also by developmental
totipotency. Until recently, the only teratocarcinoma stem-
cell sources capable of yielding all somatic tissues as well
as functional germ cells, after injection into blastocysts,
were two *in vivo* transplant lines, one chromosomally male
(X/Y) and one female (X/X); these generated germ-line progeny
in some mosaic phenotypic males and females, respectively
(Mintz and Illmensee, 1975; Cronmiller and Mintz, 1978).

We have now been able to surmount this difficulty by estab-
lishing a cell culture line with the desired properties (Mintz
and Cronmiller, 1981). The line originated from a tumour produced by the method (Stevens, 1970) of transplanting an embryo
to an ectopic site under the testis capsule, where embryogenesis becomes disorganized and early stem cells can persist.
The grafted embryo from which the cell line arose was for-
tuitously X/X. The cell line has been designated METT-1 (the
first Mouse Euploid Totipotent Teratocarcinoma cell line)
(Mintz and Cronmiller, 1981).

The developmental potential of these stem cells (of the
129 strain) was assayed by microinjecting them into blastocysts of the C57BL/6 strain (Stewart and Mintz, 1981). Biochemical markers documented the capacity of tumour-lineage
cells to contribute to formation of all somatic tissues and
to remain normal. Of ten mosaic-coat females that were test-
mated to males of the blastocyst (recessive-colour) strain,
two have produced some offspring of the diagnostic tumour-

strain agouti-colour; F_1 heterozygotes in turn transmitted
their tumour-strain genes to F_2 homozygous segregants (Stewart
and Mintz, 1981; Stewart and Mintz, 1982). The METT-1 line of
teratocarcinoma stem cells therefore bridges the gap between
the soma and germ line, and between propagation and genetic
manipulation of cells *in vitro* and embryogenesis *in vivo*.

INTRODUCTION OF FOREIGN GENE SEQUENCES INTO MICE VIA THE FERTILIZED EGG

The first successful attempt to introduce foreign DNA into a
mammal was carried out by microinjection of purified simian
virus 40 (SV40) DNA into the cavity of mouse blastocysts
(Jaenisch and Mintz, 1974), by means of micromanipulation
techniques introduced (for other purposes) by Lin (1966). The
purpose of our study (Jaenisch and Mintz, 1974) was to investigate the mechanism of incorporation of tumour viral genetic
material, its vertical transmission, and its possible activation. The DNA from some of the tissues in approximately 40%
of the resultant mice contained SV40-specific DNA sequences,
as judged from reannealing kinetics in molecular hybridization
tests with a radiolabelled SV40 DNA probe.

Those experiments were carried out before the availability
of recombinant DNA. As a result of recombinant DNA technology,
it is now possible to introduce any cloned gene in intact or
specifically modified form. Injection into the fertilized
egg might be expected to increase the number of tissues in
which the donor genetic material would be found. Synthesis
of endogenous DNA occurs in the male and female pronuclei before they fuse (Mintz, 1965b), and this pronucleate stage provides a convenient and promising stage for injection of DNA
before cleavage.

The DNA used in our first series of injections (E. Wagner
et al., 1981) included the human β-globin gene (Fritsch *et.
al.*, 1980), which would be expected to have tissue-specific
expression in erythroid cells, and the herpes simplex viral
(HSV) thymidine kinase (*tk*) gene, which would be constitutively expressed. Both genes were ligated in the same pBR322
plasmid vector, designated PtkHβ1 (obtained from T. Maniatis).
Into this vector had been spliced, at the corresponding res-
triction-endonuclease sites, the 7.6-kilobase (kb) *Hind*III
fragment of the human adult genomic β-globin gene (including
the entire gene plus approximately 6 kb of flanking sequences)
and the 3.6-kb *Bam*HI fragment of the HSV *tk* gene. Approximately 2500 copies were injected into the male (larger) pronucleus; the eggs, after brief reincubation *in vitro*, were
surgically transferred to the oviducts of pseudopregnant
females. Of 33 animals examined in late foetal stages, the

high-molecular-weight DNA of five individuals (15%), and of their placentas, was positive for the foreign globin and *tk* genes and also for pBR322 sequences. This was seen after the DNAs were digested with the designated restriction enzyme, electrophoresed in agarose gel, transferred to nitrocellulose filters (Southern, 1975), tested for hybridization with the appropriate ^{32}P-labelled restriction fragment of the respective genes, and autoradiographed. The five positive foetal-placental pairs contained 3-50 copies per cell of the human β-globin gene, of which the 4.4-kb *Pst*I diagnostic fragment spans the coding region, and 3-20 copies per cell of the 3.6-kb *Bam*HI fragment of the HSV *tk* gene (E. Wagner *et al.*, 1981).

Both the globin and *tk* genes are represented in intact copies and, in some individuals, also in higher molecular weight DNA fragments. These larger fragments probably arise as a result of changes such as deletions and duplications. Such rearrangements could involve breakage and loss of at least one specific restriction site and utilization of a cor-responding cleavage site in adjacent host DNA. Thus, the evidence is consistent with the integration of the foreign sequences into endogenous chromosomal DNA. Further data in support of this conclusion were obtained: undigested DNA did not yield any hybridizable bands corresponding to the free DNA of the plasmid, and digestion with *Sal*I, which cuts only once in this plasmid, yielded hybridizable sequences, most of which were in a broad high molecular weight band, plus some poorly separated bands, as would be expected if integration of the foreign DNA had in fact occurred at various *Sal*I sites in the host DNA (E. Wagner *et al.*, 1981).

Subsequent studies of postnatal mice from eggs injected with DNA from the same plasmid have identified animals in which donor gene sequences have persisted into adult life in stable form in all tissues tested. Transmission of donor sequences through the germ line to a fraction of the progeny has also been found and testifies to their integration in host DNA (Stewart *et al.*, 1982).

Tests were carried out on the five prenatal animals that were positive for the HSV *tk* gene to determine whether the gene was functioning to produce the HSV-type *tk* enzyme. One unequivocally positive case was identified, (E. Wagner *et al.*, 1981). The initial test was based on differences in substrate specificity of HSV and mouse enzymes; the result was confirmed in an independent test involving enzyme neutralization with antiserum specifically directed against the HSV-type enzyme. Thus, the donor gene was functional *in vivo*, even in the absence of any selective pressure or experimental induction. (No tests for the protein product of the donor globin gene

were conducted in the prenatal series; two tested postnatal
individuals were negative.)

Successful introduction and apparent integration and germ-
line transmission of recombinant DNA from other species into
mice, after injection into eggs, have also recently been reported for the intact rabbit β-globin gene (Costantini and
Lacy, 1981), the HSV *tk* gene that was fused to the promoter
of the mouse metallothionein gene(Brinster *et al.*, 1981), and
some SV40, HSV *tk*, and human interferon sequences (Gordon and
Ruddle, 1981). In another report on injection of the rabbit
β-globin gene (T. Wagner *et al.*, 1981), some evidence of
rabbit gene expression was presented. However, a Southern
blot analysis of the DNA was carried out for only one experimental mouse and revealed only internal hybridizing fragments
of the probe; there was no indication of changes in the flanking regions, of the sort that might indicate the presence of
integrated, rather than free, DNA of the donor type.

Although experiments with introduction of recombinant DNA
into mouse eggs are still in an early phase, they are promising
insofar as some expression of a constitutive gene has already
been achieved. It is possible that integration in a favourable
chromosomal site may play a major role in the usefulness of
this approach for analysing tissue-specific expression of
genes.

It is also likely that integration of any foreign gene
sequences may result in mutagenesis of host chromosomal DNA.
A change in phenotype might then enable a developmentally
regulated host gene to become analysable at the molecular
level. The phenotypic change might result in a biochemical
disease, a morphogenetic change, or even neoplastic transformation.

REFERENCES

Brinster, R.L. (1974). *J. Exp. Med.* 140, 1049-1056.
Brinster, R.L., Chen, H.Y., Trumbauer, M., Senear, A.W.,
    Warren, R. and Palmiter, R.D. (1981). *Cell* 27, 223-231.
Costantini, F. and Lacy, E. (1981). *Nature* 294, 92-94.
Cronmiller, C. and Mintz, B. (1978). *Devel. Biol.* 67, 465-
    477.
Dewey, M.J., Martin, D.W.Jr., Martin, G.R. and Mintz, B,
    (1977). *Proc. Natl. Acad. Sci. USA* 74, 5564-5568.
Fritsch, E.F., Lawn, R.M. and Maniatis, T. (1980). *Cell* 19,
    959-972.
Goldstein, J.L., Brown, M.S., Krieger, M., Anderson, R.G.W.
    and Mintz, B. (1979). *Proc. Natl. Acad. Sci. USA* 76,
    2843-2847.
Gordon, J.W. and Ruddle, F.H. (1981). *Science* 214, 1244-1246.

Gropp, A. (1975). *Clin. Genet.* 8, 389.
Jaenisch, R. and Mintz, B. (1974). *Proc. Natl. Acad. Sci. USA* 71, 1250-1254.
Karin, M. and Mintz, B. (1981). *J. Biol. Chem.* 256, 3245-3252.
Kleinsmith, L.J. and Pierce, G.B. Jr. (1964). *Cancer Res.* 24, 1544-1551.
Lesch, M. and Nyhan, W.L. (1964). *Am. J. Med.* 36, 561-570.
Lin, T.P. (1966). *Science* 151, 333-337.
Markert, C.L. (1968). *Cancer Res.* 28, 1908-1914.
Mintz, B. (1965a). *Science* 148, 1232-1233.
Mintz, B. (1965b). *In* "Ciba Foundation Symposium on Pre-implantation Stages of Pregnancy" (Eds. G.E.W. Wolstenholme and M. O'Connor), pp.145-155. J. & A. Churchill, London.
Mintz, B. (1974). *Ann. Rev. Genet.* 8, 411-470.
Mintz, B. (1978a). *Harvey Lect. Ser.* 71, 193-246.
Mintz, B. (1978b). *In* "Cell Differentiation and Neoplasia" (Ed. G.F. Saunders), pp.27-53. Raven Press, New York.
Mintz, B. (1979). *Differentiation* 13, 25-27.
Mintz, B. and Cronmiller, C. (1981). *Somatic Cell Genet.* 7, 489-505.
Mintz, B. and Fleischman, R.A. (1981). *In* "Advances in Cancer Research" (Eds. S. Weinhouse and G. Klein), Vol.34, pp.211-278. Academic Press, New York.
Mintz, B. and Illmensee, K. (1975). *Proc. Natl. Acad. Sci. USA* 72, 3585-3589.
Mintz, B., Cronmiller, C. and Custer, R.P. (1978). *Proc. Natl. Acad. Sci. USA* 75, 2834-2838.
Mulligan, R.C. and Berg, P. (1980). *Science* 209, 1422-1427.
Mulligan, R.C. and Berg, P. (1981). *Proc. Natl. Acad. Sci. USA* 78, 2072-2076.
Papaioannou, V.E., McBurney, M.W., Gardner, R.L. and Evans, M.J. (1975). *Nature* 258, 70-73.
Pellicer, A., Wagner, E.F., El Kareh, A., Dewey, M.J., Reuser, A.J., Silverstein, S., Axel, R. and Mintz, B. (1980). *Proc. Natl. Acad. Sci. USA* 77, 2098-2102.
Pierce, G.B. (1967). *In* "Current Topics in Developmental Biology" (Eds. A.A. Moscona and A. Monroy), Vol.2, pp.223-246. Academic Press, New York.
Reuser, A.J.J. and Mintz, B. (1979). *Somatic Cell Genet.* 5, 781-792.
Robins, D.M., Ripley, S., Henderson, A.S. and Axel, R. (1981). *Cell* 23, 29-39.
Seegmiller, J.E., Rosenbloom, F.M. and Kelly, W.N. (1967). *Science* 155, 1682-1684.
Southern, E.M. (1975). *J. Mol. Biol.* 98, 503-517.
Stevens, L.C. (1967). *Adv. Morphog.* 6, 1-31.
Stevens, L.C. (1970). *Devel. Biol.* 21, 364-382.

Stewart, T.A. and Mintz, B. (1981). *Proc. Natl. Acad. Sci. USA* 78, 6314-6318.

Stewart, T.A. and Mintz, B. (1982). *J. Exp. Zool.* 224, 465-469.

Stewart, T.A., Wagner, E.F. and Mintz, B. (1982). *Science* 217, 1046-1048.

Wagner, E.F. and Mintz, B. (1982). *Mol. Cell. Biol.* 2, 190-198.

Wagner, E.F., Stewart, T.A. and Mintz, B. (1981). *Proc. Natl. Acad. Sci. USA* 78, 5016-5020.

Wagner, T.E., Hoppe, P.C., Jollick, J.D., Scholl, D.R., Hodinka, R.L. and Gault, J.B. (1981). *Proc. Natl. Acad. Sci. USA* 78, 6376-6380.

Watanabe, T., Dewey, M.J. and Mintz, B. (1978). *Proc. Natl. Acad. Sci. USA* 75, 5113-5117.

Wigler, M., Silverstein, S., Lee, L.-S., Pellicer, A., Cheng, Y.-C. and Axel, R. (1977). *Cell* 11, 223-232.

Wigler, M., Pellicer, A., Silverstein, S. and Axel, R. (1978). *Cell* 14, 725-731.

PERICELLULAR MATRIX CHANGES IN FIBROBLASTIC AND EPITHELIAL CELLS INDUCED BY ONCOGENIC TRANSFORMATION

J. Keski-Oja, K. Alitalo, S. Barlati*, and A. Vaheri

*Department of Virology, University of Helsinki,
00290 Helsinki 29, Finland
*Institute of Biology, University of Brescia,
25100 Brescia, Italy*

INTRODUCTION

Cellular transformation, a model for studies on malignant growth behaviour, is characterized by a variety of changes in cellular biology. The variability of the biochemical and behavioural alterations observed in different types of cells is contrasted by a limited number of viral and cellular onco-genes (Bishop, 1982). This indicates a need for some unifying concepts.

Carcinomas are the most common neoplasms of man. Cell lines from a number of different carcinomas have been established but a major drawback remains, namely the lack of nontumourigenic control cultures. Most studies on malignant transformation have been carried out using mesenchymal cells, and many of them with rodent cell lines that are just a few steps from being malignantly transformed. It appears therefore relevant, in studies on transformation-associated phenotypic changes of cultured cells, to require the identification of the presumed oncogene(s) responsible for transformation.

Neoplastic transformation of nontumourigenic cells by chemi-cal carcinogens in culture is the result of a cascade of events initiated by the carcinogen. Several cell divisions are re-quired before transformed cells emerge from a small fraction of treated cells. The fraction of carcinogen-treated cells that eventually become neoplastic can be strongly enhanced by tumour promoters in a process termed "two-stage carcinogenesis" (Berwald and Sachs, 1963; Diamond *et al.*, 1980; Goertler *et al.*,

THEORIES AND MODELS
IN CELLULAR TRANSFORMATION

1979; Knowles and Franks, 1977). Two-stage carcinogenesis *in vitro* has been demonstrated for a fibroblastic murine cell line (Mondal and Heidelberger, 1976; Mondal *et al.*, 1976). More recently, Colburn *et al.* (1979) have also used mouse epidermal cells that were carried for 30 to 40 subcultures before individual clonal lines were derived that differed in their response to tumour promoters. Clonal lines, which responded with stable malignant transformation to treatment with biologically active phorbol esters, were considered to be "spontaneously" initiated cells and produced endogenous murine leukaemia virus (MuLV).

A long latency period between the treatment with a carcinogen/mutagen and the expression of the neoplastic phenotype is generally observed with both fibroblastic and epithelial cells. This phenomenon has been the subject of several speculations on the nature of the initiating lesion. Echols (1981) has suggested that initiating agents might induce SOS functions, known from prokaryotic cells, that involve both DNA repair as well as a genetic variation component. The action of a tumour promoter would then be to induce cellular transforming genes, and this highly induced level of expression would be fixed by the action of SOS functions.

The essential event in malignant transformation by a retrovirus is the activation of a cellular or cell derived, virus transduced *onc* gene (Hayward *et al.*, 1981; Neel *et al.*, 1981; Payne *et al.*, 1981). There is accumulating evidence that malignant transformation induced by chemical or physical agents may similarly lead to the activation of individual cellular *onc* genes (Cooper *et al.*, 1980; Shih *et al.*, 1979; Shilo and Weinberg, 1981), either directly or with endogenous retrovirus as an intermediate.

PERCELLULAR MATRIX AND TRANSFORMATION

Transformation of fibroblastic cells with oncogenic viruses have been reported to induce changes both in the pericellular matrix and in cell surface glycoproteins (Alitalo and Vaheri, 1982; Ruoslahti *et al.*, 1981; Vaheri *et al.*, 1984; Yamada and Olden, 1978). The loss of pericellular fibronectin-procollagen matrix has been a characteristic feature in almost all virally transformed cell cultures studied (see below). Loss of the noncollagenous matrix glycoprotein, laminin, from virally transformed cells (including epithelial cells) has recently been demonstrated (Alitalo *et al.*, 1982; Hayman *et al.*, 1981). It has also been reported that viral transformation of chick fibroblasts leads to a decrease in their collagen synthesis (Green *et al.*, 1966; Kamine and Rubin, 1977; Sandmeyer and Bornstein, 1979).

Post-translational modifications of collagen have been described in avian sarcoma virus-transformed cells (Myllylä *et al.*, 1981). Both chemical and viral transformation can change the collagen phenotype of cultured mesenchyme-derived cells (Hata and Peterkofsky, 1977), suggesting that the stage of differentiation has changed. The phenotype of type I procollagen was changed in fibroblastic cells transformed by oncogenic viruses and chemical carcinogens (Hata and Peterkofsky, 1977). The cells produced, after transformation, procollagen type I composed of trimers of proα1 chains. Several laboratories have reported production by normal cells of a collagen composed of three identical chains which appear to be structurally related to the α1 chain of type I collagen (c.f. Alitalo and Vaheri, 1981). Crouch and Bornstein (1978) described production of both normal type I procollagen and procollagen α1 (I) trimers by human amniotic epithelial cells suggesting that the relative production of these two related proteins may be modulated *in vitro*. In studies on MSV- and MuLV-transformed mouse epithelial cells, we found evidence of altered deposition of procollagen type I chains in the cell layers (Keski-Oja *et al.*, 1982a). The phenotype of type I procollagen thus seems to be an indicator for the transformed state of certain transformed cells.

Virus-transformed fibroblastic cells are known to produce fibronectin (Hayman *et al.*, 1981; Vaheri and Ruoslahti, 1975), in some cases less than their nontransformed counterparts (Vaheri and Ruoslahti, 1975). Epithelial cells also produce fibronectin in culture (Alitalo *et al.*, 1980 and 1981; Quaroni *et al.*, 1978; Smith *et al.*, 1979), and certain virus-transformed epithelial cells produce enhanced amounts of fibronectin into their media (see below). Studies on metastatic human carcinoma cell lines in culture have suggested that they deposit only low levels of fibronectin into their pericellular matrices, whereas cell lines derived from primary carcinomas had bundles of matrix fibronectin (Smith *et al.*, 1979). Understanding of the molecular events and the disturbances involved in the production of the matrix components and in the formation of the pericellular matrix would expand our knowledge of the role of the matrix for different types of cells.

Transformed cells frequently produce growth factors that can affect the growth properties of nontransformed cells (De Larco and Todaro, 1978). Production of plasminogen activators and type IV collagenase is often observed (c.f. Vaheri and Alitalo, 1981). Malignant epithelial cells, however, do not in general produce major amounts of plasminogen activators into their growth medium (c.f. Franks and Wigley, 1979). Therefore, the loss of the matrix may be linked to the production of plasminogen activators or to other factors undiscovered thus far.

COMPOSITION AND FUNCTIONS OF THE PERICELLULAR MATRICES

Extracellular matrices surround cells *in vivo* and two kinds
of matrices have been defined. Interstitial type connective
tissue matrix is formed in tissues between and around similar
types of cells whereas basement membranes are formed between
similar and dissimilar cells (c.f. Alitalo and Vaheri, 1982;
Vaheri *et al.*, 1983). For example, vascular basement membranes are found between connective tissues and endothelial
cells.

The pericellular matrix of cultured cells contains both
collagenous and noncollagenous protein components and glycos-
aminoglycans. The major matrix proteins identified thus far
are collagens, fibronectin and laminin (Table 1).

TABLE 1
Components of Extracellular Matrices

Interstitial	Basement membrane
Collagen types I,II,III	Collagen types IV,V,EC
Fibronectin	Fibronectin (peripheral)
Tropoelastin-elastin	Laminin
140 kd glycoprotein	Entactin
Proteoglycan	Proteoglycan

For references see Alitalo and Vaheri (1982) and Vaheri *et al.*
(1983).

Interactions between the individual matrix components have
been demonstrated between fibronectin and collagen (Engvall
et al., 1978; Dessau *et al.*, 1978), fibronectin and heparan
sulphate (Laterra *et al.*, 1980; Ruoslahti and Engvall, 1980),
aggregated cellular fibronectin and hyaluronic acid (Laterra
and Culp, 1982), sulphated gycosaminoglycans and collagen
(Öbrink, 1973), and heparan sulphate and laminin (Sakashita
et al., 1980), but all these interactions are relatively weak.
In the pericellular matrix of cultured fibroblasts sulphated
proteoglycans appear to be bound to matrix proteins by strong
non-covalent linkages (Hedman *et al.*, 1982).

Overall, the composition of the matrix surrounding the
cells is closely dependent on the cell type and the degree
of its differentiation. The composition of the matrix is

well preserved in cell culture, even after prolonged cultivation. A major function of the matrix is apparently to give
mechanical support to the cells and anchor them in tissue-type
specific structures, and possibly to function as a selective
permeability barrier. It is evident that changed or defective
cell surface-pericellular matrix interactions are salient features of the malignant phenotype.

MATRIX CHANGES IN TRANSFORMED FIBROBLAST CULTURES

Quantitatively, the most significant alteration among the
various effects of transformation of cultured fibroblastic
cells is the loss of the pericellular matrix. The loss of the
matrix was observed independently in several laboratories
using cells surface labelling and immunological techniques
(Gahmberg *et al.*, 1974; Hynes, 1973; Vaheri and Ruoslahti,
1974). Loss of the pericellular matrix upon transformation
was originally observed in a variety of cells transformed
either by viruses, spontaneously, or chemically. It was later
demonstrated that the biosynthesis (Levinson *et al.*, 1975) and
deposition (Vaheri *et al.*, 1978b) of collagen was decreased in
virus-transformed fibroblasts. Now it is known that the loss
of pericellular fibronectin is accompanied by a concomitant
loss of other matrix components (c.f. Alitalo and Vaheri,
1982). The importance of viral oncogene products in the loss
of the pericellular matrix has been established using virus
mutants temperature sensitive for transformation (Gahmberg *et
al.*, 1974; Vaheri and Ruoslahti, 1974; Hynes and Wyke, 1975;
Adams *et al.*, 1977; Arbogast *et al.*, 1977; Alitalo *et al.*,
1982).

In some transformed cells the biosynthesis of fibronectin
is drastically decreased. The major defect seems, however,
to be the inability of the transformed cells to deposit the
matrix components into extracellular structures. Although
transformation results in various modifications of the different matrix components, fibronectin, procollagen (increased
hydroxylation of prolyl and lysyl residues and glycosylation
of the latter) and heparan sulfate proteoglycan (altered
degree of sulphation), it is unclear how these alterations in
matrix molecules are responsible for the failure to deposit
them in a matrix form (see Alitalo and Vaheri, 1982). The
loss of the matrix is an essential feature of the transformed
morphology. The transformed cells will transiently acquire a
more normal phenotype if exogenous fibronectin is added into
their culture media (Yamada *et al.*, 1976a and b) or if transformed cells are grown on top of isolated cell-free fibroblast
matrices (Vaheri *et al.*, 1978a).

The loss of the pericellular matrix in transformation of

chick fibroblasts by Rous sarcoma virus (v-*src* oncogene) can
partly result from the reduction in the biosynthesis of both
fibronectin and procollagen (Adams *et al.*, 1977; Howard *et al.*,
1978; Rowe *et al.*, 1978; Fagan *et al.*, 1979 and 1981; Sandmeyer
and Bornstein, 1979; Sandmeyer *et al.*, 1981; Parker and Fitschen, 1980). The quality of the matrix proteins is also
affected. There is a quantitative change in glycosylation and
phosphorylation and also increased degradation fibronectin in
transformed cultures (Olden and Yamada, 1977; Teng and Rifkin,
1979; Ali and Hunter, 1981; Wagner *et al.*, 1981). Aberrant
sulfation of fibronectin has also been reported in cultures of
melanoma cells (Wilson *et al.*, 1981). The principal change is,
as mentioned above, that malignantly transformed mesenchymal
cells have a reduced ability to deposit the fibronectin molecules they synthesize (Vaheri and Ruoslahti, 1975; Vaheri *et
al.*, 1978b). In heterokaryons of normal and transformed
fibroblasts the transformed genotype determined the lack of
surface expression of fibronectin (Laurila *et al.*, 1979).

Dexamethasone and certain other corticoid hormones are able
to restore the fibronectin-procollagen matrix to transformed
cell cultures (Furcht *et al.*, 1979). Butyrate was also able
to induce matrix fibronectin in virus-transformed cell cultures
(Hayman *et al.*, 1980). Cultivation of cells in the presence
of these drugs restored the matrix apparently by increasing
the deposition of all matrix components in the cell layers.

PERICELLULAR MATRIX AND MALIGNANT EPITHELIAL CELLS

Studies on the biochemical alterations involved in viral transformation of epithelial cells have been hampered by the lack
of pure host cultures of nontumourigenic epithelial cells.
Most studies carried out thus far have been performed with
cultured rat liver epithelial cells or malignant cell lines
established from tumours (Borek, 1972; Knowles and Franks,
1977; Weinstein *et al.*, 1975). The biology of carcinomas
differs considerably from that of sarcomas (cf. Franks and
Wigley, 1979; Weinstein *et al.*, 1975). Identification of
changes in oncogenic transformation of cultured epithelial
cells may elucidate aspects of regulation of epithelial cell
growth and maturation.

Epithelial cells are more often exposed to different carcinogens and viruses than connective tissue cells. When epithelial cells become malignant they will penetrate through
their basement membranes and surrounding connective tissues
in order to infiltrate and metastasize. In this process they
use the capabilities induced in the cells by cellular or viral
oncogenes. The studies carried out on the structure of the
extracellular matrices in culture have shed some light on the

behaviour of normal and transformed cells *in vivo*.

Pericellular matrix appears to be essential for the maintenance of the phenotype of epithelial cell. The production and deposition of the matrix components has been studied in cultures of malignantly transformed epithelial cell lines and carcinoma cell lines established from tumours. No clear relationships have been found between the production of a specific component (e.g. fibronectin) and tumourigenicity or metastatic capacity. In spite of the fact that a number of different carcinoma cell lines have been established, there are only a few models where the comparison between nontumourigenic control cells and their malignantly transformed counterparts is appropriate.

Studies on viral transformation of cultured epithelial cells have demonstrated a different alternative in malignant phenotypes. An epithelial rat cell line has been transformed with a T-class ts-mutant of RSV (carrying the v-*src* oncogene). In these cells concomitant loss of the different pericellular matrix components (laminin, fibronectin, procollagen, heparan sulfate proteoglycan) was observed at the temperature permissive for transformation (Alitalo *et al.*, 1982). Similar observations were made when untransformed and RSV-transformed rat kidney epithelial cells were compared (Hayman *et al.*, 1981 and 1982).

As a part of studies on the nature of cellular genes involved in epithelial cell transformation, we have transformed epithelial cells in culture with murine leukaemia virus (Rapp and Keski-Oja, 1982), murine sarcoma virus (Rapp *et al.*, 1979), and with a direct-acting chemical carcinogen ethylnitrosourea. A comparison of the phenotypes of independently isolated epithelial cell transformants induced by the different agents was used as an attempt to determine whether malignant transformation of a given cell type occurs along a preferred route or whether there are multiple independent pathways for the transformation of the same cell. Epithelial cells transformed with Moloney murine sarcoma virus, (carrying the v-*mos* oncogene) or with a murine leukaemia virus, were found to secrete increased amounts of fibronectin into their growth media, but also deposited pericellular matrices containing fibronectin, procollagens, and laminin into pericellular structures (Keski-Oja *et al.*, 1982a). In contrast, another mouse sarcoma virus (3611-MSV), containing the v-*raf* oncogene, induced loss of the matrix, inhibited collagen biosynthesis, and even increased fibronectin production into the culture medium (Keski-Oja *et al.*, 1982b).

Normal epithelial cells in culture produce and deposit fibronectin into their pericellular matrices (Vaheri *et al.*, 1984). We have found that the production of fibronectin into

the medium was enhanced in certain transformed epithelial cell
cultures. MSV- and MuLV-transformed epithelial cells were,
however, able to retain pericellular fibronectin-containing
structures, and the loss of the matrix, typical of transformed
fibroblastic cells, could not be observed (Keski-Oja *et al.*,
1982a). Malignant human mammary epithelial cells were observed to produce quantities of fibronectin comparable to
those produced by control cells but the deposition in the cell
layer was deficient (Taylor-Papadimitrou *et al.*, 1981).

Thus, under certain circumstances virus-induced malignant
transformation of epithelial cells is accompanied by the loss
of the matrix, mimicking the outcome in viral transformation
of fibroblasts, but the loss is not a prerequisite for the
malignant phenotype. When the pericellular matrix is lost,
morphological cell transformation is more prominent and cell
anchorage is affected.

PROTEOLYSIS OF MATRIX COMPONENTS INDUCED BY ONCOGENIC TRANSFORMATION

Malignantly transformed and tumour derived cell lines, as
well as certain types of normal cells produce proteolytic enzymes which participate in various physiological and patho-
logical events *in vivo* such as cell invasion and migration,
and tissue destruction. The best known proteinases associated
with the transformed state are plasminogen activators (Reich,
1975) and basement membrane collagenase (Liotta *et al.*, 1979).
Liotta and others (1979) showed the existence in murine tumour
tissue of a metalloprotease with a specificity for basement
membrane collagen. In murine melanoma cell lines with varying
metastatic potential, this enzyme activity correlated with the
ability of the cells to metastasize (Liotta *et al.*, 1980).
The plasminogen activating system has quantitatively a remarkable capacity. After activation from plasminogen, plasmin has
a broad substrate specificity and it can activate, for example,
latent collagenase with interstitial or basement specificities
(Stricklin *et al.*, 1977; Moscatelli *et al.*, 1980; Liotta *et
al.*, 1981a and b). The secretion of plasminogen activators is
not restricted to the malignant phenotype but is considered a
part of the general physiological regulatory system.

Enzymatic digestion of pericellular matrix components
yields biologically active degradation products. The proteolytic fragments of the multifunctional protein, fibronectin,
have been of special interest. The ability of fibronectin
fragments to promote morphological cell transformation
(transformation-enhancing factor, TEF) was detected in cultures of fibroblasts infected with a temperature-sensitive
mutant of Rous sarcoma virus (De Petro *et al.*, 1981). TEF

activity was obtained from plasminolytic fragments of human plasma fibronectin or from cathepsin G-treated fibronectin. No TEF activity was observed in intact dimeric or reduced and alkylated fibronectin. All activity resided in the gelatin-binding fragment, which was active at nanomolar concentrations. Fibrinogen, its plasmolytic digests, or plasma transglutaminase, tested as potential contaminants of the fibronectin preparations, had no TEF activity. The TEF activity of fibronectin digests could be blocked by gelatin, excess of intact fibronectin (De Petro *et al.*, 1981), or by fibronectin antibodies (De Petro *et al.*, 1983). The small doses of the gelatin-binding fragments needed for TEF activity might suggest involvement of hormone-type or enzymatic mechanisms of action.

Whether the gelatin-binding fibronectin fragments are themselves responsible for the TEF activity or whether they act as cofactors or carriers for other components is not settled. In fact, evidence is accumulating that plasminogen activator may also be involved (De Petro *et al.*, 1984). Interestingly, the tumour promoter, TPA, shows TEF activity in the bioassay, and TEF activity is produced to the culture medium of transformed cells (Kryceve *et al.*, 1976; Kryceve-Martinerie *et al.*, 1981). These findings raised the intriguing possibility that fibronectin fragments might have an active role in morphological cell transformation.

Plasminogen activators appear to act directly on substrate(s) other than plasminogen and these effects appear to be involved in viral cell transformation as was found by using plasminogen activator-specific protease inhibitors (Quigley, 1979). Human fibrosarcoma cells have been reported to secrete proteolytic factor(s) that can affect pericellular matrix fibronectin of normal fibroblasts (Keski-Oja and Todaro, 1980). When cell-free preparations of fibroblast matrices were exposed to this factor a cleavage of a matrix-associated 66,000-dalton polypeptide and a concomitant generation of a 62,000-dalton polypeptide was seen (Keski-Oja and Todaro, 1980). Thrombin, which cleaves fibronectin at high concentrations, stimulates the release of pericellular fibronectin in intact form from cultured fibroblasts (Mosher and Vaheri, 1978). Release of fibronectin from cell-free fibroblast matrices takes place also in association with the cleavage of the 66,000-dalton protein by thrombin (Keski-Oja *et al.*, 1981) and purified urokinase (Keski-Oja and Vaheri, 1982). The 66,000-dalton protein thus appears to be a target for different proteinases and may also be associated with the release of fibronectin from the pericellular matrix.

Invasion process involves enzymatic degradation of connective tissue components, especially type IV collagen (Liotta *et al.*, 1980) and tumour-associated proteolytic fragmentation

of fibronectin may prove an indicator for tumour progression.
When tumour cells during metastasis encounter the subendothelial matrix, their ability to adhere may be needed for metastatic spread. The metastatic potential of cultured melanoma
cells appears to be related to preferential adherence to the
subendothelial matrix (Kramer *et al.*, 1981), a process possibly mediated by fibronectin (Nicolson *et al.*, 1981). Malignant cells evidently need to change their growth behaviour
during the different stages of metastasis, their interactions
with matrix components in cell anchorage, detachment and
matrix penetration.

TRANSFORMING GROWTH FACTORS AND THE MATRIX

Transforming growth factors (TGFs) are a group of polypeptides
that have the ability to induce anchorage-independent growth
of normal cells. TGFs were first observed in the culture
media of virus-transformed fibroblasts (De Larco and Todaro,
1978) and later a number of TGFs have been isolated from different cell lines. There appear to be differences in the
TGFs isolated from cells and their culture media. Some TGFs
are dependent on the presence of epidermal growth factor (EGF)
or EGF-like TGFs to fully express their effects (Anzano *et al.*,
1982). TGFs have also been observed in some normal tissues
and it is possible that the amount of some normally expressed
TGFs are enhanced and some transformation-specific TGFs are
induced (Roberts *et al.*, 1981). A new aspect on the role of
growth factors was found when homologies were observed in the
amino acid sequence of platelet-derived growth factor and the
putative transforming protein of simian sarcoma virus (Waterfield *et al.*, 1983).

TGFs are able to induce growth stimulation and focus formation in normal cell cultures (De Larco and Todaro, 1978).
These changes in the growth behaviour are evidently associated
with disturbances in the cell-matrix interactions. Thus far
the degradation of the matrix as a result of the production
of TGFs has not been possible to study. The expression of
active oncogenes and their protein products in transformed
cells as well as different TGFs will be an interesting field.

CELL ANCHORAGE AND ACTION OF ONCOGENES

The closest and evidently strongest type of adhesion of cultured cells to solid surfaces occurs through pad-like form-
ations at the ventral cell surfaces, called focal adhesions.
They are formed at the cell periphery after initial adhesion
onto the growth substratum, and considerable spreading begins
to take place. Bundles of microfilaments terminate at these

adhesions and the focal adhesions close to the cell margin appear to be devoid of pericellular fibronectin (Birchmeier *et al.*, 1980; Chen and Singer, 1980; Fox *et al.*, 1980) at least in growing cultures. In stationary cultures fibronectin is then found at the focal adhesions (Singer and Paradiso, 1981). Vinculin, the 130,000-dalton intracellular protein, is specially localized to the focal adhesions (Geiger, 1979; Burridge and Feramisco, 1980). A heavily glycosylated proteinase-resistant 140,000-dalton polypeptide is also associated with the pericellular matrices of fibroblastic cells (Carter and Hakomori, 1981; Lehto *et al.*, 1980; Lehto, 1983) and it appears to be transformation-sensitive (Carter, 1982).

Transformation of fibroblasts by Rous sarcoma virus (RSV) is evidently the best known transformation model. The transforming RSV oncogene-coded protein, a 60,000-dalton phosphoprotein, $pp60^{src}$ (see Bishop, 1982) catalyzes phosphorylation of tyrosine residues in several proteins *in vitro* (see Hunter *et al.*, 1981). Several possible substrates for $pp60^{src}$ have been identified in RSV-transformed cells (see Sefton *et al.*, 1982). In many substrate-attached transformed cells, the $pp60^{src}$ protein is enriched at the membrane ruffles and intercellular junctions, and it colocalizes with vinculin at the focal adhesions present in transformed cells (Rohrschneider, 1980; Shiver and Rohrschneider, 1981). The codistribution of vinculin with $pp60^{src}$ at the focal adhesions, and the vinculin-containing rosette-like structures that appear in transformed cells (David-Pfeuty and Singer, 1980), suggest that the $pp60^{src}$ kinase phosphorylates vinculin at the focal adhesions (Rhorschneider *et al.*, 1982). Thus the activity of $pp60^{src}$ in the focal adhesions might be responsible for different phenotypic changes that take place upon transformation. The presence of $pp60^{src}$ at the focal adhesions seems to be related to the pericellular matrix. The amount of phosphotyrosine recovered in vinculin of the focal adhesion correlated best with soft-agar growth in analysis of cells transformed by a panel of partially defective RSV mutants (Rohrschneider *et al.*, 1982). These observations suggest that the substratum may provide regulatory signals for normal cells while malignant cells may be uncoupled from this regulation. Studies on the localization of the protein products of different oncogenes will expand our knowledge of their roles in the degradation of the pericellular matrices.

REFERENCES

Adams, R.D., Sobel, M.E., Howard, B.H., Olden, K., Yamada, K.M., de Crombrugghe, B. and Pastan, I. (1977). *Proc. Natl. Acad. Sci. USA* __74__, 3399-3403.

Ali, I.U. and Hunter, T. (1981). *J. Biol. Chem.* 256, 7671-7677.

Alitalo, K. and Vaheri, A. (1982). *Adv. Cancer Res.* 37, 111-158.

Alitalo, K., Kurkinen, M., Vaheri, A., Kreig, T. and Timpl, R. (1980). *Cell* 19, 1053-1062.

Alitalo, K., Keski-Oja, J. and Vaheri, A. (1981). *Int. J. Cancer* 27, 755-761.

Alitalo, K., Keski-Oja, J., Hedman, K. and Vaheri, A. (1982). *Virology* 119, 347-357.

Anzano, M.A., Roberts, A.B., Smith, J.M., Lamb, L.C. and Sporn, M.B. (1982). *Anal. Biochem.* 125, 217-224.

Arbogast, B.W., Yoshimura, M., Kefalides, N.A., Holtzer, H. and Kaji, A. (1977). *J. Biol. Chem.* 252, 8863-8868.

Berwald, Y. and Sachs, L. (1963). *Nature (London)* 200, 1182-1184.

Birchmeier, C., Kreis, T.E., Eppenberger, H.M., Winterhalter, K.H. and Birchmeier, W. (1980). *Proc. Natl. Acad. Sci. USA* 77, 4108-4112.

Bishop, J.M. (1982). *Adv. Cancer Res.* 37, 1-32.

Borek, C. (1972). *Proc. Natl. Acad. Sci. USA* 69, 956-959.

Burridge, K. and Feramisco, J. (1980). *Cell* 19, 587-595.

Carter, W.G. and Hakomori, S. (1981). *J. Biol. Chem.* 256, 6953-6960.

Carter, W.G. (1982). *J. Biol. Chem.* 257, 3249-3257.

Chen, W-T. and Singer, S.J. (1980). *Proc. Natl. Acad. Sci. USA* 77, 7318-7322.

Colburn, N.H., Former, B.F., Nelson, K.A. and Yuspa, S.H. (1979). *Nature (London)* 282, 589-591.

Crouch, E. and Bornstein, P. (1978). *Biochemistry* 17, 5499-5509.

Cooper, G.M., Okenquist, S. and Silverman, L. (1980). *Nature* 284, 418-421.

David-Pfeuty, T. and Singer, S.J. (1980). *Proc. Natl. Acad. Sci. USA* 77, 6687-6691.

De Larco, J.E. and Todaro, G.J. (1978). *Proc. Natl. Acad. Sci. USA* 75, 4001-4008.

De Petro, G., Barlati, S., Vartio, T. and Vaheri, A. (1981). *Proc. Natl. Acad. Sci. USA* 78, 4965-4969.

De Petro, G., Barlati, S., Vartio, T. and Vaheri, A. (1983). *Int. J. Cancer* 31, 157-162.

De Petro, G., Vartio, T., Salonen, E-M., Vaheri, A. and Barlati, S. (1984). *Int. J. Cancer.* in press.

Dessau, W., Adelmann, B.C. and Timpl, R. (1978). *Biochem. J.* 169, 55.

Diamond, L., O'Brien, T.G. and Baird, W. (1980). *Adv. Cancer Res.* 32, 1-74.

Echols, H. (1981). *Cell* 25, 1-2.

Engvall, E., Ruoslahti, E. and Miller, E. (1978). *J. Exp. Med.* 147, 1584.

Fagan, J.B., Yamada, K.M., de Crombrugghe, B. and Pastan, I. (1979). *Nucleic Acids Res.* 6, 3471-3480.

Fagan, J.B., Sobel, M.E., Yamada, K.M., de Crombrugghe, B. and Pastan, I. (1981). *J. Biol. Chem.* 256, 520-525.

Fox, C.H., Cottler-Fox, M.H. and Yamada, K.M. (1980). *Exp. Cell Res.* 130, 477-481.

Franks, L.M. and Wigley, C.B. (Eds.) (1979). "Neoplastic Transformation in Differentiated Epithelial Cell Systems *In Vitro*", pp.1-314. Academic Press, London.

Furcht, L.T., Mosher, D.F., Wendelschafer,Crabb, G., Woodbridge, P.A. and Foidart, J.M. (1979). *Nature (London)* 277, 393-395.

Furie, M.B. and Rifkin, D.R. (1980). *J. Biol. Chem.* 255, 3134-3140.

Gahmberg, C.G., Kiehn, D. and Hakomori, S.I. (1974). *Nature* 248, 413-415.

Geiger, B. (1979). *Cell* 18, 193-205.

Green, H., Todaro, G.J. and Goldberg, B. (1966). *Nature (London)* 209, 916-917.

Goertler, K., Loehrke, H., Schweitzer, J. and Hesse, B. (1979). *Cancer Res.* 37, 1293-1297.

Hata, R.I. and Peterkosfky, B. (1977). *Proc. Natl. Acad. Sci. USA* 74, 2933-2937.

Hayman, E.G., Engvall, E. and Ruoslahti, E. (1980). *Exp. Cell Res.* 127, 478-481.

Hayman, E.G., Engvall, E. and Ruoslahti, E. (1981). *J. Cell Biol.* 88, 352-357.

Hayman, E.G., Oldberg, A., Martin, C.R. and Ruoslahti, E. (1982). *J. Cell Biol.* 94, 28-35.

Hayward, W.S., Neel, B.G. and Astrin, S.M. (1981). *Nature (London)* 290, 475-480.

Hedman, L., Johansson, S., Vartio, T., Kjellen, L., Vaheri, A. and Höök, M. (1982). *Cell* 28, 663.

Howard, B.H., Adams, S.L., Sobel, M.E., Pastan, I. and de Crombrugghe, N. (1978). *J. Biol. Chem.* 253, 5869-5874.

Hunter, T., Sefton, B.M. and Cooper, J.A. (1981). *Cold Spring Harbor Conf. Cell Prolif.* 8, 1189-1202.

Hynes, R.O. (1973). *Proc. Natl. Acad. Sci. USA* 70, 3170-3174.

Hynes, R.O. and Wyke, J.A. (1975) *Virology* 64, 492-504.

Howard, B.H., Adams, S.L., Cobel, M.E., Pastan, I. and de Crombrugghe, B. (1978). *J. Biol. Chem.* 253, 5869-5874.

Kamine, J. and Rubin, H. (1977). *J. Cell Physiol.* 92, 1-12.

Keski-Oja, J. and Todaro, G.J. (1980). *Cancer Res.* 40, 4722-4727.

Keski-Oja, J. and Vaheri, A. (1982). *Biochim. Biophys. Acta* 720, 141-146.

Keski-Oja, J., Todaro, G.J. and Vaheri, A. (1981). *Biochim.*

Biophys. Acta 673, 323-331.

Keski-Oja, J., Gahmberg, C.G. and Alitalo, K. (1982a). *Cancer Res.* 42, 1147-1153.

Keski-Oja, J., Rapp, U.R. amd Vaheri, A. (1982b). *J. Cell Biochem.* 20, 139-148.

Knowles, M.R. and Franks, L.M. (1977). *Cancer Res.* 37, 3917-3924.

Kramer, R.H., Vogel, K.G. and Nicolson, G.L. (1981). *J. Biol. Chem.* 257, 2678-2686.

Kryceve, C., Vigier, P. and Barlati, S. (1976). *Int. J. Cancer* 17, 370-379.

Kryceve-Martinerie, C., Biquard, J.M., Lawrence, D., Vigier, P., Barlati, S. and Mignatti, P. (1981). *Virology* 112, 436-449.

Laterra, J. and Culp, L.A. (1982). *J. Biol. Chem.* 257, 719.

Laterra, J., Ansbacher, R. and Culp, L.A. (1980). *Proc. Natl. Acad. Sci. USA* 77, 6662.

Laurila, P., Wartiovaara, J. and Stenman, S. (1979). *J. Cell Biol.* 80, 118-127.

Lehto, V-P. (1983). *Exp. Cell Res.* 143, 271-286.

Lehto, V-P., Vartio, T. and Virtanen, I. (1980). *Biochem. Biophys. Res. Commun.* 95, 909-916.

Levinson, W., Bhatnagar, R.S. and Liu, T.Z. (1975). *J. Natl. Cancer Inst.* 55, 807-810.

Liotta, L.A., Abe, S., Gehron-Robey, P. and Martin, G.R. (1979). *Proc. Natl. Acad. Sci. USA* 76, 2268-2272.

Liotta, L.A., Tryggvason, K., Garbisa, S., Hart, I., Foltz, G.M. and Shafie, S. (1980). *Nature (London)* 284, 67-68.

Liotta, L.A., Goldfarb, R.H., Brundage, R., Siegal, G.P., Terranova, V. and Garbisa, S. (1981a). *Cancer Res.* 41, 4629-2636.

Liotta, L.A., Goldfarb, R.H. and Terranova, V.P. (1981b). *Biochem. Biophys. Res. Commun.* 98, 184-190.

Mondal, S. and Heidelberger, C. (1976). *Nature (London)* 260, 710-711.

Mondal, S., Brankow, D.W. and Heidelberger, C. (1976). *Cancer Res.* 36, 2254-2260.

Mosher, D.F. and Vaheri, A. (1978). *Exp. Cell Res.* 112, 323-334.

Moscatelli, F., Rifkin, D.B., Isseroff, R.R. and Jaffe, E.A. (1980). *In* "Proteases and Tumor Invasion" (Eds. P. Sträuli, A.J. Barrett and A. Baici), pp.143-152. Raven Press, New York.

Myllylä, R., Alitalo, K., Vaheri, A. and Kivirikko, K.I. (1981). *Biochem. J.* 196, 683-692.

Neel, B.G., Hayward, W.S., Robinson, H.L., Fang, J. and Astrin, S.M. (1981). *Cell* 23, 323-334.

Nicolson, G.L., Irimura, T., Gonzales, R. and Ruoslahti, E. (1981). *Exp. Cell Res.* 135, 461-465.

Öbrink, B. (1973). *Eur. J. Biochem.* 33, 387.

Olden, K. and Yamada, K.M. (1977). *Cell* 11, 957-969.

Parker, I. and Fitschen, W. (1980). *Nucleic Acids Res.* 8, 2823-2833.

Payne, G.S., Courtneidge, S.A., Crittenden, L.B., Fadly, A.M., Bishop, J.M. and Varmus, H.E. (1981). *Cell* 23, 311-322.

Quaroni, A., Isselbacher, K.J. and Ruoslahti, E. (1978). *Proc. Natl. Acad. Sci. USA* 75, 5548-5552.

Quigley, J. (1979). *Cell* 17, 131-141.

Rapp, U.R. and Keski-Oja, J. (1982). *Cancer Res.* 42, 2407-2411.

Rapp, U.R., Keski-Oja, J. and Heine, U.I. (1979). *Cancer Res.* 39, 4111-4118.

Reich, E. (1975). *In* "Proteases and Biological Control" (Eds. E. Reich, D.B. Rifkin and E. Shaw), pp.333-341. Cold Spring Harbor Lab., Cold Spring Harbor, New York.

Roberts, A.B., Anzano, M.A., Lamb, L.C., Smith, J.M. and Sporn, M.B. (1981). *Proc. Natl. Acad. Sci. USA* 78, 5339-5343.

Rohrschneider, L.R. (1980). *Proc. Natl. Acad. Sci. USA* 77, 3514-3518.

Rohrschneider, L.R., Rosok, M. and Shiver, K. (1982). *Cold Spring Harbor Symp. Quant. Biol.* 46, 953-956.

Rowe, D.W., Moen, R.C., Davidson, J.M., Byers, P.H., Bornstein, P. and Palmiter, R.D. (1978). *Biochemistry* 17, 1581-1590.

Ruoslahti, E. and Engvall, E. (1980). *Biochim. Biophys. Acta* 631, 350.

Ruoslahti, E., Engvall, E. and Hayman, E.G. (1981). *Coll. Res.* 1, 95-128.

Sakashita, S., Engvall, E. and Ruoslahti, E. (1980). *FEBS Lett.* 116, 243.

Sandmeyer, S. and Bornstein, P. (1979). *J. Biol. Chem.* 254, 4950-4953.

Sandmeyer, S., Gallis, B. and Bornstein, P. (1981). *J. Biol. Chem.* 256, 5022-5028.

Sefton, B.M., Hunter, T., Nigg, E.A., Singer, S.J. and Walter, G. (1982). *Cold Spring Harbor Symp. Quant. Biol.* 46, 939-951.

Shih, C., Shilo, B-Z., Goldfarb, M.P., Dannenberg, A. and Weinberg, R.A. (1979). *Proc. Natl. Acad. Sci. USA* 76, 5714-5718.

Shilo, B-Z. and Weinberg, R.A. (1981). *Nature (London)* 289, 607-609.

Shriver, K. and Rohrschneider, L. (1981). *J. Cell Biol.* 89, 525-535.

Singer, I.I. and Paradiso, P.R. (1981). *J. Cell Biol.* 24, 481-492.

Smith, H.S., Riggs, J.L. and Mosesson, M.W. (1979). *Cancer*

Res. 39, 4138-4144.

Stricklin, G.P., Bauer, E.A., Jeffrey, J.J. and Eisen, A.Z. (1977). *Biochemistry* 16, 1607-1615.

Taylor-Papadimitriou, J., Burchell, J. and Hurst, J. (1981). *Cancer Res.* 41, 2491-2500.

Teng, M.H. and Rifkin, D.B. (1979). *J. Cell Biol.* 80, 784-791.

Vaheri, A. and Alitalo, K. (1981). *In* "Cellular Controls in Differentiation" (Eds. C.W. Lloyd and D.A. Rees), pp.29-54, Academic Press, London.

Vaheri, A. and Ruoslahti, E. (1974). *Int. J. Cancer* 13, 579-586.

Vaheri, A. and Ruoslahti, E. (1975). *J. Exp. Med.* 142, 530-535.

Vaheri, A., Alitalo, K., Hedman, K. Keski-Oja, J., Kurkinen, M. and Wartiovaara, J. (1978a). *Ann. N.Y. Acad. Sci.* 312, 343-353.

Vaheri, A., Kurkinen, M., Lehto, V-P., Linder, E. and Timpl, R. (1978b). *Proc. Natl. Acad. Sci. USA* 75, 4944-4948.

Vaheri, A., Alitalo, K., Hedman, K., Keski-Oja, J. and Vartio, T. (1983). *In* "Structural Carbohydrates in the Liver", Falk Symposium No.34, pp. 385-398.

Vaheri, A., Keski-Oja, J. and Vartio, T. (1984). *In* "Fibronectin" (Ed. D.F. Mosher), Academic Press, New York, in press.

Wagner, D., Ivatt, R., Destree, A. and Hynes, R. (1981). *J. Biol. Chem.* 256, 11708-11715.

Waterfield, M.D., Scrace, G.T., Whittle, N., Stroobant, P., Johnsson, A., Wasteson, Å., Westermark, B., Heldin, C.-H., Huang, J.S. and Deuel, T.F. *Nature (London)* 304, 35-39.

Weinstein, I.B., Yamaguchi. N., Gebert, R. and Kaigh, E.M. *Vitro (Rockville)* 11, 130.

Wilson, B.S., Ruberto, G. and Ferrone, S. (1981). *Biochem. Biophys. Res. Commun.* 101, 1047-1051.

Yamada, K.M. and Olden, K. (1978). *Nature (London)* 275, 179-184.

Yamada, K.M., Ohanian, S.H. and Pastan, I. (1976a). *Cell* 9, 241-245.

Yamada, K.M., Yamada, S.S. and Pastan, I. (1976b). *Proc. Natl. Acad. Sci. USA* 73, 1217-1221.

MOLECULAR ASPECTS OF NGF-INDUCED ARREST OF MITOSIS AND NEURITE OUTGROWTH IN PC12 CELLS

P. Calissano[+], S. Biocca[++], A. Cattaneo[*], A. Di Luzio[+], and D. Mercanti[+]

[+]*Istituto di Biologia Cellulare C.N.R., Via G. Romagnosi, 18A Roma, Italy*
[++]*On leave of absence from the Istituto di Chimica Biologica dell'Universita di Roma, Italy*
[*]*On leave of absence from the Scuolao Normale Superiore di Pisa, Italy*

INTRODUCTION

The discovery of the polypeptide nerve growth factor (NGF) (Levi-Montalcini, 1952; Levi-Montalcini and Cohen, 1956; Levi-Montalcini and Booker, 1960) soon followed by that of epidermal growth factor (EGF) (Cohen, 1959 and 1962; for review see Carpenter and Cohen, 1979), brought to light the existence of an entirely new class of biologically active proteins and raised the problem of their functional significance and proper place in the field of developmental biology. NGF and EGF not only are the best characterized of these new hormone-like substances, but their biological actions have a direct bearing on two interrelated aspects of normal and deviant cell biology, proliferation and differentiation. Thus, while the most peculiar action of EGF is that of stimulating division of target cells, NGF plays a fundamental trophic and differentiative function on sensory and sympathetic cells (for a summary of its properties see Table 1).

More recent studies uncovered another important property of these two polypeptides, related to cell transformation. The mitogenic action exerted by EGF on target cells occurs via stimulation of phosphorylation of tyrosines in a group of proteins which are identical to those phosphorylated by some oncogenes (Hunter and Cooper, 1981; Erikson *et al.*, 1981)

TABLE 1

Properties of Nerve Growth Factor (NGF)

Denomination	βNGF; 2.5S NGF (lack of N-terminal octapeptide and C-terminal arg. with no relevance to biological action)
Structure	2 subunits of 13.250 daltons 3 intramolecular S-S bridges resistant to acids and alkali
Sources	Minute quantities (ng/mg proteins) several normal and neoplastic cells Large quantities (µg/mg ") snake venom; mouse and mastomys salivary glands; guinea pig prostate; bull seminal fluid
Target Cells	Sympathetic cells (throughout all life) Sensory and chromaffin cells (early developmental stages)
Function	Trophic: key role for survival of target cells Tropic: induction of neurite growth along its concentration gradient Phenotipic modulation: Pheochromocytoma cells ⟶ sympathetic-like cells Pheochromoblasts --------⟶ sympathetic-like cells
Mechanism of action	Receptor binding ---⟶ patching ---⟶ internalization ---⟶ retrograde axonal transport ---⟶ intracellular distribution ---⟶?

For review on NGF properties see: Levi-Montalcini (1966), Levi-Montalcini and Angeletti (1968), Mobley *et al.*, (1977), Levi-Montalcini and Calissano (1978), Bradshaw (1978), Thoenen and Barde (1980), Varon and Adler (1980), Greene and Shooter (1980), Calissano *et al.*, (1983).

TABLE 2

Temporal Dissection of NGF Effects on PC12 Cells

	Minutes	Hours	Days
		-NGF-R internalization	-Arrest of mitosis
			-Neurites outgrowth
		-Increased aminoacids and glucose transport	-Priming (RNA synthesis dependent)
	-Binding		-MTs and MFs assembly
	-Patching	-Increased ODC	-Electrical excitability
NGF-Receptors	-Membrane ruffling	-Increased adhesiveness	-Stimulation of: TTL, AchE, CAT, NILE, MAP-I
		-Stimulation Na$^+$ - K$^+$ pump	-Increased receptors for: NGF, Acetylcholine, enkefalins
			-Inhibition of 34K-ssbp

Abbreviations used: ODC = ornitine decarboxylase
TTL = Tyrosósil tubulin ligase
AchE = Acetylcholinesterase
CAT = Choline acetyltransferase
NILE = NGF-inducible-large-external
MT = Microtubule; MF = Microfilament
34K-ssbp = single-strand DNA binding protein

73

suggesting that the same basic mechanism may transduce both a normal (EGF) and abnormal (oncogene) signal of cell division. On the other hand, the differentiative action exerted by NGF is most dramatically evidenced in a clonal cell line (PC12) derived from a rat pheochromocytoma tumor (Greene and Tischler, 1976; Dichter *et al.* 1977; Greene and Shooter, 1980). In these cells NGF not only exerts its typical differentiative action characterized by induction of neurite outgrowth but it also causes these cells to cease dividing as a prerequisite of the former effect (a temporal dissection of NGF effects upon these cells is reported in Table 2).

This multiple, impressive response of PC12, as well as their nature of neoplastic clonal cell line, called the attention of several investigators, attracted not only by the possibility of analysing the mechanism of action of NGF but also of studying, under strictly controlled conditions, the molecular steps accompanying the differentiation of a neoplastic cell into its neuronal counterpart.

Ever since early reports on the action of NGF on PC12 cells (Greene and Tischler, 1976) our laboratory has been engaged in analysing some steps of the response of these cells to this growth factor. In particular, we have focused our efforts on two molecular systems: the NGF receptor (s) and the cytoskeleton, with special reference to microtubules (MTs) and microfilaments (MFs). The former as the most obvious candidate to play a central role in transducing the NGF message, the latter as the universally acknowledged network mediating neurite outgrowth and elongation which represents the most impressive morphological response of target cells to NGF.

We shall summarize these studies and present some new findings related to the possible mechanism through which NGF exerts another crucial action i.e. arrest of PC12 division.

RESULTS

The NGF Receptor(s)

In PC12 cells there are $3-5 \times 10^4$ specific NGF binding sites/cell which increase seven- to ten-fold on a per cell basis during onset of morphological differentiation induced by NGF (Calissano and Shelanski, 1980; Cattaneo *et al.*, 1983). An aliquot of these sites are located on axons and dendrites as indicated by autoradiographic studies. It is not yet clear whether increase in NGF receptors in NGF-treated PC12 cells is the consequence of exposure of an intracellular pool or, more probably, expression of neosynthesis of those proteins (e.g activation of a biosynthetic pathway for those proteins (e.g.

tubulin and actin) essential for neurite outgrowth and elongation. As it will be reported below, PC12 cells do indeed
possess a pool of hidden receptors (Cattaneo *et al.*, 1983) but
their possible contribution to the increase observed in NGF-
treated PC12 cells is negligible since they constitute 40-50%
of the total originally present in naive cells which possess
only 1/7 - 1/10 of the site number detected in NGF-treated cells.
Binding of ^{125}I.NGF to these cells is rapidly followed by
internalization of NGF-receptor complexes as indicated by disappearance of receptors on the cell surface (Calissano and
Shelanski, 1980; Biocca *et al.*, 1980) and concomitant intra-
cellular accumulation of labelled NGF and NGF-antibodies cross-
reacting material within certain cellular compartments (Marchisio *et al.*, 1980). Disappearance of NGF receptors following
exposure of naive PC12 to the ligand, also known as down regulation, is evidenced when cells are not confluent and does not
occur at confluency, suggesting a possible modulation of NGF
effect as a function of cell density (Biocca *et al.*, 1980).
This possibility has been further stressed by the demonstration
that priming of PC12 cells (Greene and Shooter, 1980), the process
through which these cells acquire the property of responding
much faster to this factor on a second presentation, is better
evidenced when cells are incubated with NGF at low density,
i.e. when down regulation of NGF receptor complexes occurs.
This correlation suggests that the pool of internalized NGF-
receptors may play an important role in priming of PC12 cells.
Massive, synchronous internalization of NGF is achieved within
4-8 h incubation and occurs only upon the first exposure of
this factor (Biocca *et al.*, 1980). This process reaches subsequently a sort of steady state (Layer and Shooter, 1983)
whereby the number of NGF molecules entering the cell is
counterbalanced by degradation of an approximate equal number,
so that the net total labelled cellular NGF remains constant
and increases slowly every day (as reported above) with the
onset of morphological differentiation, due to increase in
cell size and receptor-bearing neurites.
    The pool of internalized NGF is detectable within the cyto-
plasm and around the nuclear membrane under the form of discrete dots (Marchisio *et al.*, 1980); the presence of a small
pool in a perinucleolar contour is still not unequivocally
proved (Marchisio *et al.*, 1980; Bernd and Greene, 1983).
    A controversial aspect of NGF receptors is whether they
are formed by a single, homogeneous population or whether in
PC12 cells there are at least two distinct classes. This
question was raised by the finding that at 37°C NGF bound to
its receptors exhibits different dissociation rates (Landreth
and Shooter, 1980). Kinetic studies of NGF interaction with
its receptor(s) performed at 37°C are complicated by the

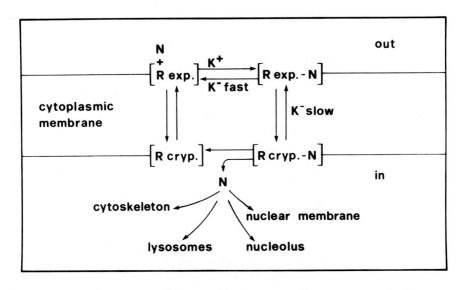

FIG. 1 *Dynamics of NGF–receptors interaction. Free NGF (N)
binds to receptors (R-exp) exposed on the external surface
of the plasma membrane of PC12 cells. The NGF-receptor complexes (R-exp-N) may either dissociate and mimick low affinity
receptors or become cryptic (R-cryp) and behave as slow dissociating high affinity sites. These hidden NGF-receptor complexes may either reappear on the external surface or undergo
internalization and distribute intracellularly (as evidenced
by autoradiographic, immunofluorescence and electron microscopic studies) as depicted by the arrows in the figure. The
question mark underlines the indirect evidence about cito-
skeletal distribution of a portion of internalized NGF, which
has been obtained on fixed and permeabilized cells incubated
with NGF (Nasi et al., 1982).*

subsequent fate of the complexes which undergo patching (Levi
et al., 1980) and internalization (Calissano and Shelanski,
1980). At low temperatures (Herrup and Thoenen, 1979) or in
cells whose dynamic state is blocked by metabolic poisoning or
paraformaldehyde fixation (Cattaneo *et al.*, 1983) NGF receptors
behave as a single, kinetically homogeneous population with a
Kd of 2.7 x 10^{-9}M. The latter studies also revealed that a
fraction of 40-50% of total NGF receptors are buried within
the membrane, inaccessible to NGF or to trypsin digestion.
This pool of hidden receptors can rapidly exchange with those
exposed on the cell surface independently from the presence of
NGF. These findings would be in favour of the hypothesis
(Cattaneo *et al.*, 1983) that the prospected "heterogeneity" of
NGF receptors is due to different location (exposed or hidden)
of the same population rather than expression of distinct
molecular species. According to this view the pool of NGF
bound to receptors present on the external surface (see Fig. 1)
may either rapidly exchange with free NGF molecules (mimicking
fast dissociating, low affinity sites) or may participate in
the fate of another pool of receptors and become cryptic, thus
exhibiting a much slower dissociation rate and higher affinity.
In this connection it is worth recalling that other receptor
systems have been shown to undergo recycling even in the
absence of the ligand (Brown *et al.*, 1983). The discovery of
the existence of two pools of NGF receptors has suggested
their involvement in the chemotactic response of growing neurites to NGF (Gundersen and Barrett, 1979) as a mechanism to
"sense" the gradient of concentration of the surrounding molecules (Cattaneo *et al.*, 1983).

Cytoskeletal Elements in the NGF-mediated Neurite Outgrowth

As previously remarked (Calissano *et al.*, 1976) the cytoskeleton and in particular its more dynamic elements, microtubules (MTs) and microfilaments (MFs), act as the intra-
cellular "transmission belt" of NGF action. Their function
is that of transducing chemical energy into mechanical work
which is utilized by each cell according to its special need.
Neurons, besides employing MTs and MFs for the common cellular
functions (dynamics of chromosomes and other organelles, lat-
eral diffusion of membrane proteins etc.) depend upon these
cytoskeletal structures for growth and branching of neurites.
    Modulation of MTs and MFs assembly and function can be
achieved by different mechanisms such as control of local
concentrations of Ca^{++}, or nucleotides such as ATP and GTP,
or via the action of a group of proteins operationally defined
as MT and MF associated proteins (MAPs, MFPs). The MAPs and
MFPs modulate assembly of precursors elements (tubulin and

actin), link MTs to other cellular components or cross-link MFs
with each other to form gels and sols (for review see Goldman
et al., 1976; Timasheff and Grisham, 1980).

MTs and MFs are comparable to "modular elements regulated
in their specific performances by specific proteins expressed
by different cells according to their special need and function" (Calissano *et al.*, 1976). On the basis of these considerations it has been hypothesized that NGF modulates the
synthesis or the post-translational modifications of some MAPs
within the context of its action in promoting massive and fast
generation or regeneration of meurites. This growth factor
has in fact been recently shown to increase the synthesis of
a >300.000 m.w. phosphoprotein in PC12 cells which, on the
basis of different criteria, has been considered a sub-species
of a high molecular weight, microtubules associated protein
(Greene *et al.*, 1983). Moreover, cellular extracts derived
from fully differentiated PC12 cells (PC12+) stimulate assembly
of exogenously added purified tubulin (Biocca *et al.*, 1983).
This stimulatory effect was identified in a macromolecular
moiety sedimenting at 100.000 x g (but not at 80.000) and
defined as 100 K x g pellet. The same structure is also present in naive PC12 cells (PC12-) but it contains much lower
amounts of 3 proteins of m.w. 100K, 88K and 34K. This activity
promoting tubulin assembly is destroyed by detergent treatment
or preincubation of PC12+ cells with colchicine. Indirect
evidence, to be corroborated by further studies (*in vitro* reconstitution of this macromolecular structure and identification of the component(s) responsible for its supramolecular
organization) suggests that some of the proteins selectively
enriched in PC12+ cells confer to the 100 K x g pellet a tri-
dimensional organization more suitable to promote MTs assembly.

Molecular Aspects of NGF-induced Mitotic Arrest

Mitotic arrest and neurite outgrowth induced by NGF in PC12
cells occur slowly and are fully achieved only after two to
three weeks incubation with this growth factor. These two
fundamental cellular events presumably occur in a synchronous
fashion, so that only those cells which have turned off their
molecular system for DNA duplication and cell division will
activate the protein network (cytoskeleton) which causes the
cell to change shape and to grow axons and dendrites.

In the previous section we have reported studies aimed at
identifying proteins whose synthesis is turned on by NGF in
relation to this latter event; in this section we will shortly
present evidence that NGF turns off the synthesis of a protein which may play a central role in the process of DNA
duplication. These studies started when an analysis of the

proteins co-assembling with microtubules and forming the
100 K x g pellet (see previous section) responsible for the
increased rate of assembly of purified brain tubulin, showed
a marked reduction of a 34 K dalton protein of basic charge
(Biocca *et al.*, 1983). Initial speculations brought us to
attribute to this protein a role of inhibitor of MT assembly
and to associate its progressive disappearance during onset
of neurite outgrowth with increased polymerization of MTs
necessary for axonal elongation. However, an analysis in prokaryotes of the proteins directly implicated in DNA replication
(Alberts and Grey, 1970; Kornberg, 1980) revealed the existence
of a polypeptide endowed with the property of unwinding DNA,
in advance of DNA-polymerase activity, which share m.w. and
charge with the 34 K dalton protein identified in our studies.
This structural similarity, and the consideration that its
synthesis was progressively suppressed with arrest of PC12
cell division and decreased thymidine incorporation caused by
NGF, suggested to us its possible homology with the protein(s)
identified in prokaryotes. This hypothesis received unequivo-
cable validation by the use of double stranded (ds) and single
stranded (ss) DNA colums on which ^{35}S-labelled cellular extracts derived from PC12- and PC12+ cells were chromatographed
(Biocca *et al.*, 1984). Thus, one peculiar property of these
types of proteins, generally known as unwinding, helix de-
stabilizing or single strand DNA binding proteins is that they
bind to denatured but not to native, double stranded DNA.
These experiments demonstrated that the 34K protein progressively disappearing in PC12 cells under NGF action binds to
ss-DNA but not to ds-DNA and that use of this purification
protocol allows, with a single step, to obtain this protein in
an almost pure form (Fig. 2). Subsequent studies demonstrated
that it constitutes 0.5 - 1.0% of total soluble proteins, that
a pool of this polypeptide is (∿15%) phosphorylated and that
it exists, under non-denaturing conditions, as an oligomer
probably made of four, 34 K dalton subunits. Turnover studies
indicate that it has a half-life (∿90 h) much longer than that
of other cellular proteins (52 h) and that its synthesis is
even more rapidly suppressed by concomitant incubation of PC12
cells with NGF and mitotic inhibitors of different nature such
as OH-urea, cytosine arabinoside, colchicine and taxol. Although the function of this protein in PC12 cells remains to
be ascertained, its direct involvement in DNA replication or
in other functions such as transcription, recombination etc
appears highly probable in view of its unique affinity for
ss-DNA and considering that suppression of its synthesis co-
incides with cellular events where DNA must play a central
role.

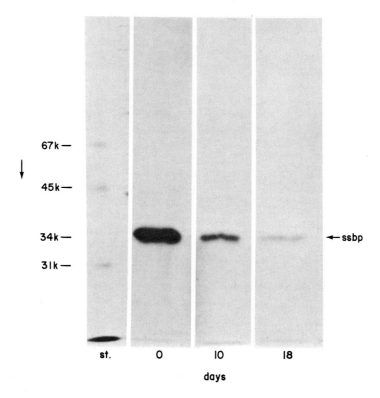

FIG. 2 *Inhibition of the synthesis of the 34K-ssb protein
under NGF action. Autoradiogram after SDS-acrylamide gel
electrophoresis of the 34K-ssb protein isolated from a
100.000 x g supernatant of ^{35}S-labelled cellular extracts
derived from PC12 cells incubated without NGF (day 0) or with
this factor for 10 and 18 days. The arrow indicates the protein, which can be obtained in an almost pure form with only
one ss-DNA chromatography. Notice the progressive decrease
of the labelled protein following incubation with NGF.*

DISCUSSION

In order to explore the mechanism of action of NGF we resorted
to a particularly favourable model system (PC12 cells) whereby
the many effects of this factor can be analysed under suitable
experimental conditions. It was our main goal to identify
the molecular system(s) which, on a theoretical and experimental ground, must play a <u>direct role</u> in mediating the response to NGF action. These are, as reported in this article,
i) the receptor(s), ii) the cytoskeleton and iii) the proteins
involved in DNA function and replication. We realize that

each of this set of proteins is endowed with a great complexity and is subjected to multiple modulatory elements. However, only a coordinated molecular approach can uncover the chain of events directly involved in NGF action as a first step in the elucidation of its mode of action.

As already mentioned in the previous section these sets of proteins must be somewhat linked so as to respond in a synchronous fashion to a signal which, alone, results in the effect of mitotic arrest and activation of a differentiative programme. This dual function can be exerted in parallel, with, for instance, a receptor mediated reorganization of cytoskeletal elements at the level of the plasma membrane (where these filaments are anchored) and at the nuclear level through the agency of the internalized pool of NGF-receptor complexes. Alternatively, the NGF effect can occur in series whereby modulation of the function of the cytoskeleton results not only in outgrowing of neurites but also in the arrest of cell division via some as yet unidentified communication system between cytoskeletal elements and the nuclear compartment (Folkmann and Moscona, 1978; Ben Ze'ev et al., 1980; Wittelsberg et al., 1981). Within the context of this second hypothesis one should also consider the possibility of a direct intervention of NGF on MTs and on MFs as demonstrated to occur in vitro in a cell-free system (Calissano and Cozzari, 1974; Calissano et al., 1978).

Whatever the correct explanation, it is clear that in order to achieve its multiple effects NGF must regulate these molecular systems via control of the synthesis or postranslational modifications of "modulatory proteins". Our studies have identified some of these polypeptides, respectively implicated in control of MTs assembly and of DNA replication or function. In particular, the 34K-ssb protein may play a crucial role in maintaining PC12 cells in their transformed state and suppression of its synthesis by NGF may constitute a conditio-sine-qua-non for their differentiation in a sympathetic-like cell population.

ACKNOWLEDGEMENTS

We wish to thank Dr R. Levi-Montalcini for stimulating discussion and criticism during the preparation of this manuscript.

This work has been supported in part with a grant no. 204121/96/93256, "Progetto Finalizzato Controllo della Crescita Neoplastica" from C.N.R. to P. Calissano and with grant no. 1-848 March of Disues.

REFERENCES

Alberts, B. and Frey, L.M. (1970). *Nature* 227, 1313-1316.

Ben Ze'ev, A., Farmer, S.R. and Penmann, S. (1980). *Cell* 21, 365-372.

Bernd, D. and Greene, L.A. (1983). *J. Neurosci.* 3, 631-643.

Biocca, S., Levi, A. and Calissano, P. (1980). *J. Receptor Research* 1, 373-387.

Biocca, S., Cattaneo, A. and Calissano, P. (1983). *EMBO J.* 2, 643-648.

Biocca, S., Cattaneo, A. and Calisanno, P. (1984). *Proc. Natl. Acad. Sci.* in press.

Bradshaw, R.A. (1978). *Ann. Rev. Biochem.* 47, 191-216.

Brown, M.S., Anderson, R.G.W. and Goldstein, J.L. (1983). *Cell* 32, 663-667.

Calissano, P. and Cozzari, C. (1974). *Proc. Natl. Acad. Sci. USA* 71, 2131-2135.

Calissano, P. and Shelanski, M.L. (1980). *Neuroscience* 5, 1033-1039.

Calissano, P., Levi, A., Alemà, S., Chen, S.J. and Levi-Montalcini, R. (1976). *In* "Molecular Basis of Motility" (Eds. L.M.G. Heilmeyer, J.C. Ruegg and T.H. Weiland), pp.186-200, Springer Verlag, Berlin.

Calissano, P., Monaco, G., Castellani, L., Mercanti, D. and Levi, A. (1978). *Proc. Natl. Aca-. Sci. USA* 75, 2210-2215.

Calissano, P., Cattaneo, A., Aloe, L. and Levi-Montalcini, R. (1984). *In* "Hormonal Proteins and Peptides", Vol.12, Edited by C.H. Li. Academic Press. In press.

Carpenter, G. and Cohen, S. (1979). *Ann. Rev. Biochem.* 48, 193-216.

Cattaneo, A., Biocca, S., Nasi, S. and Calissano, P. (1983). *Eur. J. Biochem.* 135, 285-290.

Cohen, S. (1959). *J. Biol. Chem.* 234, 1129-1135.

Cohen, S. (1962). *J. Biol. Chem.* 237, 1555-1562.

Dichter, M.A., Tischler, A.S. and Greene, L.A. (1977). *Nature* 268, 501-504.

Erikson, E., Shealy, P.J. and Erikson, R.L. (1981). *J. Biol. Chem.* 256, 11381-11385.

Folkman, J. and Moscona, A. (1978). *Nature* 273, 345-349.

Greene, L.A. and Tischler, A.S. (1976). *Proc. Natl. Acad. Sci. USA.* 73, 2424-2428.

Greene, L.A. and Shooter, E.M. (1980). *Ann. Rev. Neurosci.* 3, 353-402.

Greene, L.A., Liem, R.K.H. and Shelanski, M.L. (1983). *J. Cell. Biol.* 96, 76-83.

Herrup, K. and Thoenen, H. (1979). *Exp. Cell Res.* 121, 71-78.

Hunter, T. and Cooper, S.A. (1981). *Cell* 24, 741-750.

Kornberg, A. (1980). "DNA Replication", W.H. Freeman and Company, San Francisco.

Landreth, G. and Shooter, E.M. (1980). *Proc. Natl. Acad. Sci. USA* 77, 4751-4755.

Layer, P.G. and Shooter, E.M. (1983). *J. Biol. Chem.* 258, 3012-3018.

Levi, A., Schechter, Y., Neufeld, E.J. and Schlessinger, J. (1980). *Proc. Natl. Acad. Sci. USA* 77, 3463-3473.

Levi-Montalcini, R. (1952). *Ann. N.Y. Acad. Sci.* 55, 330-343.

Levi-Montalcini, R. (1966). *Harvey Lecture* 60, 217-259.

Levi-Montalcini, R. and Angeletti, P.U. (1968). *Physiol. Rev.* 48, 534-569.

Levi-Montalcini, R. and Booker, B. (1960a). *Proc. Natl. Acad. Sci. USA* 46, 373-384.

Levi-Montalcini, R. and Booker, B. (1960b). *Proc. Natl. Acad. Sci. USA* 46, 384-391.

Levi-Montalcini, R. and Calissano, P. (1978). *Scientific American* 240, 68-77.

Levi-Montalcini, R. and Cohen, S. (1956). *Proc. Natl. Acad. Sci. USA* 42, 695-699.

Marchisio, P.C., Naldini, L. and Calissano, P. (1980). *Proc. Natl. Acad. Sci. USA* 77, 1656-1660.

Mobley, W.C., Server, A.C., Ishi, D.N., Riopelle, R.J. and Shooter, E.M. (1977). *New Engl. J. Med.* 297, 1096-1218.

Nasi, S., Cirillo, D., Naldini, L., Marchisio, P.C. and Calissano, P. (1982). *Proc. Natl. Acad. Sci. USA* 79, 820-824.

Thoenen, H. and Barde, Y.A. (1980). *Physiol. Rev.* 6, 1284-1335.

Timasheff, S.N. and Grisham, L.M. (1980). *Ann. Rev. Biochem.* 49, 565-591.

Varon, S. and Adler, R. (1980). *In* "Current Topics in Developmental Biology" (Eds. A. Moscona and A. Monroy), Vol.XVI, pp.206-251.

Wittelsberger, S.C., Kleene, K. and Penman, S. (1981). *Cell* 24, 859-866.

HUMAN T-CELL LEUKAEMIA VIRUSES AND ONCOGENES AND THE ORIGIN OF SOME HUMAN LEUKAEMIAS AND LYMPHOMAS

R.C. Gallo, F. Wong-Staal, M.F. Clarke, H-G. Guo, E. Westin, W.C.Saxinger, W.A. Blattner and M.S. Reitz, Jr.

Laboratory of Tumor Cell Biology, Family Studies Section, National Cancer Institute, National Institutes of Health, Bethesda, Maryland 20205, USA

INTRODUCTION

Retroviruses are etiological agents of naturally occurring leukaemias and lymphomas in many animal species (for review see Gallo and Wong-Staal, 1980). For this reason they are known as leukaemia viruses. Some are acutely transforming, and these retroviruses carry transformation specific genes (*onc* genes) derived from highly conserved normal cellular genes (c-*onc*) that may be important in basic cellular functions and/or differentiation (Bishop, 1978). In recent years it has been shown that these genes are also present in humans (for review see Wong-Staal and Gallo, 1982). Other retroviruses are chronic leukaemia viruses, and some of these have been shown to cause leukaemia by activating c-*onc* genes (Hayward, Neel and Astrin, 1981; Neel *et al.*, 1981). We have two major interests in retroviruses: (1) Using the acutely transforming animal retroviruses as "tools", one can detect, isolate, and analyse c-*onc* genes in human DNA in order to help clarify the basic abnormalities in the growth and/or differentiation of human blood cells found in the leukaemias and lymphomas. (2) Since chronic leukaemia viruses are an important cause of naturally occurring leukaemias and lymphomas of many animals, these retroviruses have been sought almost since the beginning of this century as a possible cause of these diseases in humans. Here we describe recent results from our laboratory in both these areas of retrovirus research.

THEORIES AND MODELS
IN CELLULAR TRANSFORMATION

HUMAN c-*onc* GENES

We have molecularly cloned into λ phage genomic DNA clones for the human c-*onc* genes which are homologous to the transforming genes of simian sarcoma virus (SSV-sis) (Dalla Favera *et al.*, 1981), feline sarcoma virus (FeSV-*fes*) (Franchini *et al.*, 1982), avian myelocytomatosis virus (MC29-*myc*) (Dalla Favera *et al.*, 1982d), and avian myeloblastosis virus (AMV-*myb*) (Franchini *et al.*, submitted). All human cellular *onc* genes contain sequences homologous to the entire viral *onc* genes, as well as extra coding regions not present in their viral counterparts, but these are interrupted by nonhomologous introns varying in lengths and number. In addition, several *myc*-related pseudogenes characterized by their incompleteness, lack of introns and greater divergence from v-*myc* have been analysed (Dalla Favera *et al.*, 1982d). In collaboration with C. Croce we have mapped the chromosomal localization of several human *onc* genes (Dalla Favera *et al.*, 1982b; 1982c; Harper *et al.*, 1983). These are shown in Table 1. One of them, c-*myc* is of particular interest. It is located on the distal end of the long

TABLE 1

Chromosomal Location of Some Human onc *Genes*

Onc gene	Chromosome	Other Genes on Same Chromosome
Myb	6	HLA complex
Myc	8	–
Fes	15	β2 microglobulin
Sis	22	λ chain of immunoglobulin

arm of chromosome 8. We have found that it is translocated to chromosome 14 (usually) or to chromosome 2 or 22 (seldom) in Burkitt's lymphoma (Dalla Favera *et al.*, 1982a) and in some other poorly differentiated human B-cell lymphomas (Dalla Favera *et al.*, 1982e). The translocation is into immunoglobulin gene regions, and in many cases the sequences adjacent to *myc* are rearranged. In an acute promyelocytic leukaemia cell line (HL60), which we established from a woman with this disease, we found abundant transcription of the c-*myc* gene, and this increased level of c-*myc* RNA is correlated with a 20 to 30-fold amplification of this gene in the primary (fresh cells) as well as in the cultured HL60 cells (Dalla Favera *et al.*, 1982e). These leukaemic cells can be induced to terminally differentiate to mature granulocytes with characteristics of normal cells and we have recently shown that with this induction to differentiate the c-*myc* gene is "turned off" (Westin *et al.*, 1982). These studies suggest that c-*myc* may be important in the genesis of some human leukaemias and lymphomas.

We have also examined a wide spectrum of human cells of neoplastic and normal origin for expression of other c-*onc* genes. The results showed that certain genes are almost universally transcribed while others show more specificity with respect to tissue type, lineage, or stages of differentiation. With the possible exception of expression of c-*sis* in glioblastoma and sarcoma cell lines (Eva *et al.*, 1982), we do not find the expression of any of the tested *onc* genes to be highly correlated with specific neoplasias.

HUMAN T-CELL LEUKAEMIA/LYMPHOMA VIRUS

The list of leukaemia viruses now includes a human retrovirus, called human T-cell leukaemia/lymphoma virus or HTLV. This virus was first isolated in our laboratory repeatedly from T-cell leukaemia and lymphoma cells of some American adult patients (Poiesz *et al.*, 1980a; Poiesz *et al.*, 1981; Reitz *et al.*, 1981; Gallo *et al.*, 1982). These isolates were made possible by the growth of these cells in culture with a protein we discovered in 1975 which was released into the media by activated, mature, human fresh T-lymphocytes of the helper/inducer class (Morgan *et al.*, 1976; Ruscetti *et al.*, 1977). This protein, called T-cell growth factor (TCGF), also called Il-2, promotes growth of other mature T-cells after they are activated by appropriate antigens because only then do normal T-cells develop TCGF receptors. T-cells from adults with HTLV associated leukaemias and lymphomas, however, respond directly to TCGF. They have TCGF receptors without *in vitro* antigen stimulation (Poiesz *et al.*, 1980b).

HTLV is a novel, exogenous, horizontally transmitted type-C retrovirus (Reitz *et al.*, 1981; Kalyanaraman *et al.*, 1981; Robert-Guroff *et al.*, 1981). Seroepidemiological studies, as shown in Table 2, reveal a strong and specific association of HTLV with certain types of mature T-cell malignancies of adults, including but not restricted to Japanese adult T-cell leukaemia, lymphosarcoma cell leukaemia among West Indian populations, certain other non-Hodgkins lymphomas in the same group, and peripheral T-cell lymphomas (diffuse large or mixed cell lymphomas) in various parts of the world (Catovsky *et al.*, 1982; Kalyanaraman *et al.*, 1982a; Robert-Guroff *et al.*, 1982; Blattner *et al.*, 1982; Gallo *et al.*, 1983a; Blayney *et al.*, 1983).

TABLE 2

Prevalence of Natural Antibodies to HTLV in Sera of Patients with Malignancies of Mature T-cells, their Healthy Relatives, and Random Normal Donors

Serum Donors	Antibodies to HTLV	
	No. Positive/No. Tested	% Positive
Healthy relatives of US patients with HTLV-associated malignancy	2/12	17
Unrelated healthy donors, Washington, D.C.	1/185	<1
Unrelated healthy donors, Georgia	3/158	2
Caribbean T-LCL patients	11/11	100
Healthy relatives of Caribbean patients	3/16	19
Random healthy donors, Caribbean	12/337	4
Japanese ATL patients	40/46	87
Healthy relatives of ATL patients	19/40	48
Random healthy donors, non-endemic area	9/600	2
Random healthy donors, endemic area	50/419	12

There are now more than 20 HTLV isolates comprising two distinct groups obtained from patients from many parts of the world, including Japan, the United States, the Caribbean, and Israel (Miyoshi *et al.*, 1981a; Haynes *et al.*, 1983a; Popovic *et al.*, 1983b). As shown in Table 3, analyses of the proteins and nucleic acids of the various HTLV isolates show that most belong to a single readily definable group closely related to the first HTLV isolate (Poiesz *et al.*, 1981; Popovic *et al.*,

TABLE 3

Comparison of Properties of HTLV Isolates

Designation	Cell Line	Geographic origin	RNA	p24	p19
HTLV-I$_{CR}$	HUT102	US	*	*	*
HTLV-I$_{MJ}$	MJ	US	++	++	++
HTLV-I$_{MB}$	CTCL-2	Caribbean	++	++	++
HTLV-I$_{MI}$	MI	Caribbean	++	++	++
HTLV-I$_{UK}$	UK	Israel	++	++	++
HTLV-I$_{SK}$	SK	Japan	ND	++	++
HTLV-I$_{TK}$	TK	Japan	ND	++	++
HTLV-I$_{HK}$	HK	Japan	ND	++	++
HTLV-I$_{SD}$	SD	Japan[†]	++	++	++
HTLV-I$_{MT-1}$ ("ATLV")	MT-1	Japan	++	++	++
HTLV-I$_{MT-2}$ ("ATLV")	MT-2	Japan	++	++	++
HTLV-II$_{MO}$	MO	US	±	+	++

* = Prototype HTLV

++ = Highly related to or indistinguishable from the prototype

± = Slightly or not significantly related

+ = Related but readily distinguishable

† = A cell line developed from a 49 year old female ATL patient born in Kyushu, Japan and emigrated to the United States at age 23.

1982; 1983). This group we call HTLV type I. One isolate
(Kalyanaraman *et al.*, 1982b) from a case of hairy cell leukaemia, T-cell variant (Golde *et al.*, 1978) is readily distinguishable from the other isolates by protein serology
(Kalyanaraman *et al.*, 1982b) and nucleic acid homology (Reitz
et al., 1983; Gelmann *et al.*, Proc. Nat. Acad. Sci. USA (in press

POSSIBLE MECHANISMS OF HTLV-INDUCED LEUKAEMOGENESIS

There are several ways in which retroviruses are thought to
be able to initiate cell transformation and hence to induce
neoplasias. As mentioned above, the acutely transforming
viruses cause rapid transformation *in vitro* due to their recombination with certain types of cellular genes (called *"onc"*
genes). The acquired *onc* genes are under control of the viral
RNA polymerase promotor present in the viral large terminal
repeat (LTR) and are thereby constitutively expressed in infected cells. Acutely transforming viruses are usually replication defective and require a helper virus. Disease induction,
like transformation *in vitro*, is rapid. In contrast, the
chronic leukaemia viruses, in which category most naturally
occurring leukaemia viruses belong, do not usually cause cell
transformation *in vitro* and induce disease only after long
latent periods. Some chronic leukaemia viruses appear to induce leukaemia by activating cellular *onc* genes as a result of
provirus integration in their immediate vicinity (Hayward,
Neel and Astrin, 1981; Neel *et al.*, 1981; Nusse and Varmus,
1982; Payne, Bishop and Varmus, 1982). The viral LTRs include
sequences which can promote or enhance RNA transcription of
DNA sequences in their vicinity, and this process has been
termed "downstream promotion". This requires integration
close to the target gene, and since retrovirus integration is
not thought to be highly specific, the fraction of integration
events which lead to *onc* activation is likely to be very low.
These two mechanisms are presented schematically in Fig. 1.

We and others have shown that infection of cord blood T-
cells with HTLV *in vitro* results in the rapid appearance of
some of the properties observed with transformed cells as well
as with tumour cells from ATL patients (Miyoshi *et al.*, 1981b;
Markham *et al.*, 1983; Popovic *et al.*, 1983a; 1983b). These
include a reduced requirement for (and sometimes independence
of) TCGF, a change in morphology, a change in surface phenotype which includes the expression of high levels of the TCGF
receptor and HLA-DR antigens and usually an $OKT4^+8^-$ phenotype,
an increased growth rate, and an abrogation of the crisis
period observed with uninfected T-cells four to five weeks
after initiation. Transformation and establishment of T-cell
lines has also been achieved by HTLV infection of adult human

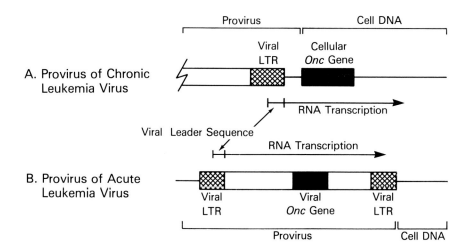

FIG. 1 *Mechanisms of cell transformation by chronic and acute leukaemia viruses. (A) The provirus from a chronic leukaemia virus integrates into the vicinity of a cellular oncogene resulting in its unregulated transcription. Only rare integrations result in transformation. (B) The provirus from an acute transforming virus integrates into the host cell genome, and carries its own oncogene with it. All integrations are potentially transforming.*

bone marrow (Markham *et al.*, 1984). The surface phenotype of these cells can be OKT4$^+$8$^-$, 4$^+$8$^+$, or 4$^-$8$^-$, apparently depending on the strain of HTLV used. These biological properties are similar to those reported for some of the acutely transforming viruses.

It is obvious, however, that like many of the animal chronic leukaemia viruses, HTLV does not always induce disease. Many normal people have persistent HTLV antibodies (Blattner *et al.*, 1982; Kalyanaraman *et al.*, 1982a; Robert-Guroff *et al.*, 1982; Schupbach *et al.*, 1983; Suchi and Tajima, 1983) or even replicating virus (Robert-Guroff *et al.*, 1983). Indeed, it has been established that, similar to the case with bovine and feline leukaemia virus, only one in 2000 antibody positive people in Japan develop ATL (Suchi and Tajima, 1983) (albeit the rate could be considerably higher in some populations). Moreover, disease appears to follow a long latent phase. These data suggest that HTLV-induced neoplasms do not involve an acutely transforming virus.

Molecular evidence that HTLV probably does not induce

A. HTLV *env-pol* probe

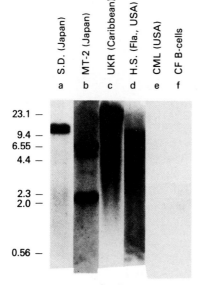

Sst I

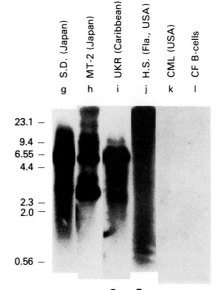

Sma I

B. HTLV LTR probe (U5-R)

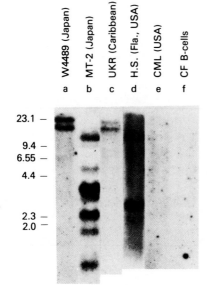

Sst I

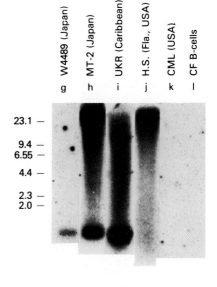

Sma I

leukaemia by means of a defective transforming virus has been
obtained using a molecular clone of HTLV recently constructed
by Manzari *et al.* (1983).   Integrated proviral sequences can
be detected by Southern blots of DNA of peripheral blood lymphocytes or cultured T-cells from persons with HTLV-associated
malignancy (Hahn *et al.*, 1983; Manzari *et al.*, 1983; Wong-
Staal *et al.*, 1983; Yoshida, Miyoshi and Hinuma, 1982).   These
Southern blots show that the DNA from the cells of each tumour
contains one or a few monoclonal integration sites; that is,
the provirus is present at precisely the same site in the DNA
of each cell.   This is exactly the same situation that has
been observed with avian and murine tumours induced by chronic
retroviruses (Hayward, 1981; Neel *et al.*, 1981; Nusse and
Varmus, 1982; Payne, Bishop and Varmus, 1982).   Since transformation by viruses which do not carry an oncogene may depend
upon integration into a specific site, since the amount of
host cell DNA is large, and since retrovirus integration is
not precise, the number of transforming events is likely to
be very low.   When the rare transforming event takes place,
the affected single cell gives rise to the tumour.   If proviral
integration sites are monoclonal, restriction endonuclease
fragments which contain both proviral and host DNA sequences
(junction fragments) will appear on Southern blots with the
same intensity as single copy genes.   In contrast, if there is
no dominant integration site, the proviral-host junction fragments are not detected or appear as faint bands or a blur on
Southern blots.   As shown in Fig. 2, using an LTR specific
probe, the former case is observed.   With all the DNA samples
shown (except for DNA from the ATL cell line MT-2), Sst I
digestion does not result in detectable internal fragments,

Legend to Fig. 2 (opposite)

FIG. 2 *HTLV proviral DNA in adult T-cell lymphomas from dif-*
ferent geographical regions. The indicated DNA was digested
with Sst I or Sma I as indicated and subjected to analysis by
Southern blotting using either an HTLV env-pol *probe (Panel A)*
or an LTR U5-R probe (Panel B). Arrows indicate the relative
positions of a marker of Hind III digested λ phage DNA. In
the Sma I digests the prominent band at 4.3 Kb (in Panel A) is
an internal fragment extending from just within the right hand
LTR to a site within pol, *while the 0.8 Kb fragment (in Panel*
B) is an internal fragment encompassing most of the left hand
LTR and a small part of the adjacent gag *region.*

since all the resultant fragments are larger than a complete
provirus and the junction bands obtained are approximately of
the intensity expected for a single copy gene. Sma I digests,
in contrast, contain internal fragments, including the 4.3 Kb
fragment visualized with an *env-pol* probe, and the 0.8 Kb
fragment seen using an LTR (U5 + R) probe. These internal
fragments are the same in all DNA samples shown except for
Sma I digests of DNA from an American patient with adult T-
cell lymphoma (H.S.) (lane j). This difference is because
this DNA sample was obtained from fresh blood cells. The
Sma I sites of the provirus are, in our experience, invariably
methylated in DNA from fresh peripheral blook leukaemic cells
and hence resistant to cleavage (M. Clarke *et al.* (in press)
whereas they are not methylated in DNA from corresponding
long-term cell lines. We have not so far been able to identify defective proviruses flanked by two LTRs, which would be
expected for a defective transforming virus. This further
suggests that HTLV does not contain a defective transforming
virus. Thus far, using the subcloned integration site from
clone CR-1 (Manzari *et al.*, 1983) as a probe, we have not
detected any common integration sites in different patients.
As other cloned proviruses become available, however, such a
site or sites may well be found.

It is possible that a retrovirus could induce genes relevant
to neoplasia by means other than downstream promotion. For
example, we have recently cloned a gene which is not associated with HTLV sequences, but which is expressed at high
levels in all HTLV-infected cell lines but not in their uninfected counterparts (Manzari *et al.*, 1982). The pattern of
expression of this gene in uninfected haemopoietic cells suggests that its expression may be linked to TCGF expression or
response, and that it may somehow be indirectly induced by
HTLV infection.

One observation made on HTLV-infected uncultured peripheral
blood leukaemic cells is that they express low to undetectable
levels of viral mRNA (Franchini *et al.*, submitted). This is
similar to what has been shown with bovine leukaemia (Kettman
et al., 1981). Upon placing these cells in culture, however,
a rapid increase occurs in viral mRNA expression (M. Clarke
et al. Virology (in press). Thus, continuous expression of
HTLV in the circulating blood cells may not be required to
maintain their leukaemic phenotype, although viral expression
in other cells may be necessary.

Another consistent observation with all HTLV infected cells
is that they express an unusual number of HLA class I allo-
typic determinants, including ones which are inappropriate to
the genetic background of the infected cells (Gallo *et al.*,
1982; Mann *et al.*, 1983). These determinants can be detected

both by microcytotixicity assays using alloantisera (Gallo
et al., 1982) and with a polymorphic monoclonal antibody
specific for the HLA-B5-15 cross-reactive group and the HLA-
A11-29-30 cross-reactive group (Mann *et al.*, 1983). Recently,
a nucleic acid homology has been reported between the *env*
gene region of HTLV and the region of an HLA class I gene
which codes for the extracellular portion of the class I antigen (Clarke, *et al.*, 1983). This homology suggests   suggests
but does not prove that the viral genome encodes the super-
numerary HLA class I specifcities. If the HTLV *env* gene indeed shares an epitope with certain class I antigens, then
perhaps the mechanism of infection involves binding of virus
to a class I antigen recognition site, which could explain its
apparent T-cell tropism. One of the *gag*-related proteins
(p19) has also been shown to be related antigenically to a
normal cellular protein present specifically on the neurendo-
crine component of uninfected human thymus (Haynes *et al.*,
1983b). Mimicry of normal cell proteins might help HTLV to
escape immune responses, or alternatively might elicit an
autoimmune response to thymic tissue. In the case of one
patient with HTLV-associated disease (who was unusual by virtue of responding to chemotherapy with a long-term survival)
it has been possible to show a cytotoxic T-cell response
which is directed towards antigens on HTLV-infected cells
(Mitsuya *et al.*, 1983). This response is HLA-restricted, and
occurs with the autologous tumour cells as well as with other
HTLV-infected tumour cells which are partly HLA-matched.

Obviously, much further work is required to begin to understand the precise ways in which HTLV exerts its apparent
leukaemogenic potential. In addition, it will be most important to determine whether HTLV is associated with diseases
other than adult T-cell malignancies. In this light, HTLV-
related viruses (Gallo *et al.*, 1983b) and viral DNA (Gelmann
et al., 1983) and antibodies (Essex *et al.*, 1983) have been
detected in a significant fraction (but not a majority) of
patients with acquired immune deficiency syndrome (AIDS).
Transmission of HTLV does not appear to be facile. Long intimate contact, such as occurs in families, and blood trans-
fusions seem to be two ways in which transmission occurs. The
various routes of transmission of HTLV, however, require
further elucidation. Answers to these and other questions
will undoubtedly be of benefit in either the prevention or
treatment of ATL and any other HTLV-related diseases, and
could even provide insight into some of the processes involved
in non-HTLV associated malignancies.

A POSSIBLE ORIGIN OF HTLV?

A possible reason for the fairly tight geographical clustering
of HTLV, other than the apparent difficulty of transmission,
is that HTLV is either a relatively new virus or has entered
the human population fairly recently. The presence of antibodies to HTLV has been noted in Japanese macaques (Miyoshi
et al., 1982). We have also observed that a substantial fraction of African green monkeys, as well as Chinese and Japanese
macaques have some serum antibodies to HTLV structural proteins
(W.C. Saxinger *et al.*, in preparation). Moreover, some of the
seropositive animals have proviral DNA specifically related to
that of $HTLV_I$ (H.G. Guo *et al.* 1984). Human serum
samples from Africa have recently shown that HTLV may be endemic to certain parts of that continent (W.A. Blattner *et
al.*, submitted).   From these results, it is interesting
to speculate that HTLV may have entered the human population
from non-human primates in Africa. The virus could then have
reached the Caribbean and surrounding regions via the slave
trade. It is also possible that HTLV could have been carried
to Japan from Africa by Portuguese adventurers. This seems
reasonable in view of the tight clustering of HTLV endemic
areas to the southwestern Japanese islands, the regions these
Europeans frequented. Whether or not this is the case, it is
obviously important to determine the extent of the current
geographic range of HTLV, and whether its range is stable or
could be increasing.

ACKNOWLEDGEMENTS

The authors wish to thank Ms Anna Mazzuca for expert editorial
assistance.

REFERENCES

Bishop, J.M. (1978). *Annu. Rev. Biochem.* 47, 35-88.
Blattner, W.A., Kalyanaraman, V.S., Robert-Gouroff, M., Lister,
    T.A., Galton, D.A.G., Sarin, P., Crawford, M.H., Catovsky,
    D., Greaves, M. and Gallo, R.C. (1982). *Int. J. Cancer*
    30, 257-264.
Blayley, D.W., Blattner, Q.A., Robert-Guroff, M., Jaffe, E.,
    Fisher, R.I., Bunn, P.A., Patton, M.G., Rarick, H.R. and
    Gallo, R.C. *J. Am. Med. Assoc.* in press.
Catovsky, D., Rose, M., Goolden, A.W.G., White, J.M., Bourikas,
    G., Brownell, A.I., Blattner, W.A., Greaves, M.F., Galton,
    D.A.G., McCluskey, D.R., Lambert, I., Ireland, R., Bridges,
    J.M. and Gallo, R.C. (1982). *Lancet* 1, 639-643.
Clarke, M., Gelmann, E.P. and Reitz, M.S. (1983). *Nature* 305,
    60-62.

Dalla Favera, R., Gelmann, E.P., Gallo, R.C. and Wong-Staal, F. (1981). *Nature* 292, 31-35.

Dalla Favera, R., Bregni, M., Erikson, S., Patterson, D., Gallo, R.C. and Croce, C.M. (1982a). *Proc. Natl. Acad. Sci. USA* 79, 7824-7827.

Dalla Favera, R., Franchini, G., Martinotti, S., Wong-Staal, F., Gallo, R.C. and Croce, C.M. (1982b). *Proc. Natl. Acad. Sci. USA* 79, 4714-4717.

Dalla Favera, R., Gallo, R.C., Giallongo, A. and Croce, C. (1982c). *Science* 218, 686-688.

Dalla Favera, R., Gelmann, E.P., Martinotti, S., Franchini, G., Papas, T.S., Gallo, R.C. and Wong-Staal, F. (1982d). *Proc. Natl. Acad. Sci. USA* 79, 6497-6501.

Dalla Favera, R., Wong-Staal, F. and Gallo, R.C. (1982c). *Nature* 299, 61-63.

Dalla Favera, R., Martinotti, S., Gallo, R.C., Erikson, J. and Croce, C.M. (1983). *Science* 219, 963-967.

Essex, M., McLane, M.F., Lee, T.H., Falk, L., Howe, C.W.S., Mullins, S.J., Cabradilla, C. and Francis, D.P. (1983). *Science* 220, 859-862.

Eva, A., Robbins, K.C., Andersen, P.R., Srinivasan, A., Tronick, S.R., Reddy, E.P., Ellmore, N.W., Galen, A.T., Lautenberger, J.A., Papas, T.S., Westin, E.H., Wong-Staal, F., Gallo, R.C. and Aaronson, S.A. (1982). *Nature* 295, 116-119.

Franchini, G., Gelmann, E.P., Dalla Favera, R., Gallo, R.C. and Wong-Staal, F. (1982). *Mol. Cell. Biol.* 2, 1014-1019.

Gallo, R.C. and Wong-Staal, F. (1980). *In* "Viral Oncology" (Ed. G. Klein), pp.399-431. Raven Press, New York.

Gallo, R.C., Mann, D., Broder, S., Ruscetti, F.W., Maeda, M., Kalyanaraman, V.S., Robert-Guroff, M. and Reitz, M.S. Jr. (1982). *Proc. Natl. Acad. Sci. USA* 79, 5680-5684.

Gallo, R.C., Kalyanaraman, V.S., Sarngadharan, M.G., Sliski, A., Vonderheid, E.C., Maeda, M., Yoshinobu, N., Yamada, K., Ito, Y., Gutensohn, N., Murphy, S., Bunn, P.A. Jr., Catovsky, D., Greaves, M.F., Blayney, D.W., Blattner, W., Jarrett, W.F.H., zur Hausen, H., Seligmann, M., Brouet, J.C., Haynes, B.F., Jegasothy, B.V., Jaffe, E., Cossman, J., Broder, S., Fisher, R.I., Golde, D.W. and Robert-Guroff, M. (1983a). *Cancer Res.* 43, 3892-3899.

Gallo, R.C., Sarin, P.S., Gelmann, E.P., Robert-Guroff, M., Richardson, E., Kalyanaraman, V.S., Mann, D.L., Sidhu, G.D., Stahl, R.E., Zolla-Pazner, S., Liebowitch, J. and Popovic, M. (1983b). *Science* 220, 865-867.

Gelmann, E.P., Popovic, M., Blayney, D., Masur, H., Sidhu, G., Stahl, R.E. and Gallo, R.C. (1983). *Science* 220, 865-

Golde, D.W., Quan, S.G. and Cline, M.J. (1978). *Blood* 52, 1068-1072.

Guo, H.-G., Wong-Staal, F. and Gallo, R.C. (1984). *Science* 233: 1195-1197.

Hahn, B., Manzari, V., Colombini, S., Franchini, G., Gallo, R.C. and Wong-Staal, F. (1983). *Nature* 303, 253-256.

Harper, M.E., Franchini, G., Love, J., Simon, M.C., Gallo, R.C. and Wong-Staal, F. (1983). *Nature* 304, 169-171.

Haynes, B.F., Miller, S.E., Palker, T.J., Moore, J.O., Dunn, P.H., Bolognesi, D.P. and Metzgar, R.S. (1983a). *Proc. Natl. Acad. Sci. USA* 80, 2054-2058.

Haynes, B.F., Robert-Guroff, M., Metzgar, R.S., Franchini, G., Kalyanaraman, V.S., Palker, T. and Gallo, R.C. (1983b). *J. Exp. Med.* 157, 907-920.

Hayward, W.S., Neel, B.G. and Astrin, S.M. (1981). *Nature* 290, 475-480.

Kalyanaraman, V.S., Sarngadharan, M.G., Poiesz, B.J., Ruscetti, F.W. and Gallo, R.C. (1981). *J. Virol.* 38, 906-915.

Kalyanaraman, V.S., Sarngadharan, M.G., Nakao, Y., Ito, Y., Aoki, T. and Gallo, R.C. (1982a). *Proc. Natl. Acad. Sci. USA* 79, 1653-1657.

Kalyanaraman, V.S., Sarngadharan, M.G., Robert-Guroff, M., Miyoshi, I., Blayley, D., Golde, D. and Gallo, R.C. (1982b). *Science* 218, 571-573.

Kettman, R., Marbaix, G., Mammerick, M. and Burny, A. (1981). *In* "Haematology and Blood Transfusion, Modern Trends in Human Leukaemia IV", Vol. 26, (Eds. R. Neth, R.C. Gallo, T. Graft, K. Mannweiller and K. Winkler), pp.495-497. Springer-Verlag, Berlin.

Mann, D.L., Popovic, M., Sarin, P., Murray, C., Reitz, M.S., Strong, D.M., Haynes, B.F., Gallo, R.C. and Blattner, W.A. (1983). *Nature* 305, 58-60.

Manzari, V., Gallo, R.C., Franchini, G., Westin, E., Ceccherini-Nelli, L., Popovic, M. and Wong-Staal, F. (1982). *Proc. Natl. Acad. Sci. USA* 80, 11-15.

Manzari, V., Wong-Staal, F., Franchini, G., Colombini, S., Gelmann, E.P., Oroszlan, S., Staal, S. and Gallo, R.C. (1983). *Proc. Natl. Acad. Sci. USA* 80, 1574-1578.

Markham, P.D., Salahuddin, S.Z., Kalyanaraman, V.S., Popovic, M., Sarin, P.S. and Gallo, R.C. (1983). *Int. J. Cancer* 31, 413-420.

Markham, P.D., Salahuddin, S.Z., Macchi, B., Robert-Guroff,M., and Gallo, R.C. (1984) *Int. J. Cancer* 33, 13-17.

Mitsuya, H., Matis, L.A., Megson, M., Bunn, P.A., Murray, C., Mann, D.L., Gallo, R.C. and Broder, S. (1983). *J. Exp. Med.* 158, 994-999.

Miyoshi, I., Kubonishi, I., Yoshimoto, S., Akagi, T., Ohtsuki, Y., Shiraishi, Y., Nagata, K. and Hinuma, Y. (1981a). *Nature* 294, 770-771.

Miyoshi, I., Yoshimoto, S., Kubonishi, I., Taguchi, H., Shiraishi, Y., Ohtsuki, Y. and Akagi, T. (1981b). *Gann* 72, 997-998.

Miyoshi, I., Yoshimoto, S., Fujishita, M., Taguchi, H., Kubonishi, I., Niiya, K. and Minezawa, M. (1982). *Lancet* ii, 658.

Morgan, D.A., Ruscetti, F.W. and Gallo, R.C. (1976). *Science*
   193, 1007-1008.
Neel, B.G., Hayward, W.S., Robinson, H.L., Fang, J. and Astrin,
   S.M. (1981). *Cell* 23, 323-334.
Nusse, R. and Varmus, H.E. (1982). *Cell* 31, 99-109.
Payne, G.S., Bishop, J.M. and Varmus, H.E. (1982). *Nature*
   295, 209-213.
Poiesz, B.J., Ruscetti, F.W., Gazdar, A.F., Bunn, P.A., Minna,
   J.C. and Gallo, R.C. (1980a). *Proc. Natl. Acad. Sci. USA*
   77, 7415-7419.
Poiesz, B.J., Ruscetti, F.W., Mier, J.W., Woods, A.M. and
   Gallo, R.C. (1980b). *Proc. Natl. Acad. Sci. USA* 77, 6815-
   6819.
Poiesz, B.J., Ruscetti, F.W., Reitz, M.S., Kalyanaraman, V.S.
   and Gallo, R.C. (1981). *Nature* 294, 268-271.
Popovic, M., Kalyanaraman, V.S., Sarngadharan, M.G., Robert-
   Guroff, M., Nakao, Y., Reitz, M.S., Miyoshi, Y., Ito, Y.,
   Minowada, J. and Gallo, R.C. (1982). *Nature* 300, 63-66.
Popovic, M., Lange-Wantzin, G., Sarin, P.S., Mann, D.L. and
   Gallo, R.C. (1983a). *Proc. Natl. Acad. Sci. USA* 80, 5402-
   5406.
Popovic, M., Sarin, P.S., Robert-Guroff, M., Kalyanaraman,
   V.S., Mann, D., Minowada, J. and Gallo, R.C. (1983b).
   Science 219, 856-859.
Reitz, M.S., Poiesz, B.J., Ruscetti, F.W. and Gallo, R.C.
   (1981). *Proc. Natl. Acad. Sci. USA* 78, 1887-1891.
Reitz, M.S., Popovic, M., Haynes, B., Clark, S. and Gallo,
   R.C. (1983). *Virology* 126, 688-692.
Robert-Guroff, M., Ruscetti, F.W., Posner, L.E., Poiesz, B.J.
   and Gallo, R.C. (1981). *J. Exp. Med.* 154, 1957-1964.
Robert-Guroff, M., Nakao, Y., Notake, K., Ito, Y., Sliski, A.
   and Gallo, R.C. (1982). *Science* 215, 975-978.
Robert-Guroff, M., Kalyanaraman, V.S., Blattner, W.A.,
   Popovic, M., Sarngadharan, M.G., Maeda, M., Blayney, D.,
   Catovsky, S., Bunn, P.A., Shibata, A., Nakao, Y., Ito, Y.,
   Aoki, T. and Gallo, R.C. (1983). *J. Exp. Med.* 157, 248-
   258.
Ruscetti, F.W., Morgan, D.A. and Gallo, R.C. (1977). *J.
   Immunol.* 119, 131-138.
Schupbach, J., Kalyanaraman, V.S., Sarngadharan, M.G.,
   Blattner, W.A. and Gallo, R.C. (1983). *Cancer Res.* 43,
   886-891.
Suchi, T. and Tajima, K. (in press). *In* "The Role of the
   Environment and Pathogenesis of Leukemias and Lymphomas"
   (Ed. I. Magrath. Raven Press, New York.
Westin, E.H., Wong-Staal, F., Gelmann, E.P., Dalla Favera, R.,
   Papas, T.S., Lautenberger, J.A., Eva, A., Reddy, E.P.,
   Tronick, S.R., Aaronson, S.A. and Gallo, R.C. (1982).

Proc. Natl. Acad. Sci. USA 79, 2490-2494.

Wong-Staal, F. and Gallo, R.C. (1982). *In* "Advances in Viral Oncology", Vol.1, (Ed. G. Klein), pp.153-171, Raven Press, New York.

Wong-Staal, F., Hahn, B., Manzari, M., Colombini, S., Franchini, G., Gelmann, E.P. and Gallo, R.C. (1983). *Nature* 302, 626-628.

Yoshida, M., Miyoshi, I. and Hinuma, Y. (1982). *Proc. Natl. Acad. Sci. USA* 79, 2031-2035.

MOLECULAR ASPECTS OF INDUCED DIFFERENTIATION OF TRANSFORMED CELLS WITH NON-CYTOTOXIC AGENTS

P.A. Marks, M. Sheffery and R.A. Rifkind

DeWitt Wallace Research Laboratory and the Sloan-Kettering Division, Graduate School of Medical Sciences, Memorial Sloan-Kettering Cancer Center New York, New York 10021, USA

INTRODUCTION

The nature of the molecular and cellular events involved in the transition of cells capable of self-renewal to terminally differentiated cells, with loss of capacity for cell division is one of the important, unresolved issues in biology. We have studied this problem employing murine erythroleukaemia cells (MELC) as a model system. MELC represents a relatively homogeneous population of virus transformed erythroid precusors (Marks and Rifkind, 1978). Among the properties of MELC that make them suitable for these studies is the fact that cells can be maintained for an essentially unlimited period of time under appropriate *in vitro* conditions (Friend *et al.*, 1971; Ruben *et al.*, 1976). MELC (inducer-sensitive strain 745A-DS19 was employed in all studies unless otherwise noted) can be induced by a variety of agents, including dimethylsulfoxide (Me$_2$SO) (Friend *et al.*, 1971), hexamethylene bisacetamide (HMBA) (Ruben *et al.*, 1976), butyric acid (Leder and Leder, 1975) and other agents to express characteristics of erythroid cell differentiation (Marks and Rifkind, 1978).

Induced differentiation of MELC is characterized by the coordinated expression of a developmental programme very similar to normal terminal erythroid differentiation including commitment to terminal cell division (Gusella *et al.*, 1976; Fibach *et al.*, 1977), and increased accumulation of α and β globin mRNA (Ross *et al.*, 1972; Ohta, 1976), of α, β^{maj}, β^{min} globins and haemoglobins major (Hb^{maj}) and minor (Hb^{min})

Boyer *et al.*, 1972; Ostertag *et al.*, 1972), of haeme synthes-
izing enzymes (Sassa, 1976), of membrane-associated erythroid
specific proteins, such as spectrin and glycophorin (Eisen,
1977), and a variety of other proteins including the chromatin
associated protein, H1° (Chen *et al.*, 1982; Keppel *et al.*,
1977).

A number of laboratories, including our own, have provided
data that suggest that the virally transformed MELC are blocked
at a stage in the erythroid lineage which is relatively late
in erythropoiesis, e.g. CFU-e (Fig. 1) (see Marks and Rifkind,
1978 for references). MELC are more differentiated and more
restricted in potential than pluripotent haemopoietic stem
cells. In view of the evidence that differentiation potential
in MELC is restricted primarily to the erythroid line, it is
reasonable to suggest that certain molecular events, required
to determine erythroid-specific lineage characteristics have
already occurred in MELC. On the other hand, those molecular
events which are required for the transition from CFU-e to the
full expression of terminal erythroid cell differentiation
occur only as inducer-mediated terminal differentiation proceeds.

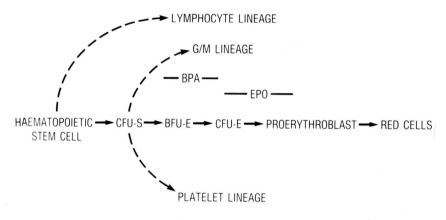

Pluripotent   **Restricted**   **Terminally Differentiated**
Precursors   **Precursors**   **Cells**

FIG. 1 *Schematic representation of sequential stages of*
haematopoietic cell development. The pluripotent precursors,
haemopoietic stem cells, produce the lymphocyte lineage and
precursors (CFU-s) of granulocyte/macrophages, erythroid cells
and platelets. Erythroid precursors, BFU-e, differentiate to
CFU-e: both are precursors of retricted potential and, in turn,
generate proerythroblasts and terminally differentiated red
cells.

COMMITMENT TO TERMINAL CELL DIVISION

Several lines of evidence suggest that commitment to terminal cell division is a multi-step process. Commitment to terminal cell division is defined as the ability of MELC to express the transition from cells capable of unlimited proliferation to terminal division (Fibach *et al.*, 1977). Inducer-mediated MELC commitment to terminal cell division exhibits different kinetics with different inducers (Nudel *et al.*, 1977; Marks *et al.*, 1979; Eisen *et al.*, 1978; Pragnell *et al.*, 1980; Chen *et al.*, 1982; Levenson and Housman, 1981; Levenson *et al.*, 1979; Marks *et al.*, 1983). Recently, our laboratories developed variants of MELC with altered patterns of response to inducers with respect to terminal cell division, including variants which failed to exhibit inducer-mediated commitment to terminal cell division, although they express other characteristics of erythroid cell differentiation (Marks *et al.*, 1983).

Work in our laboratory analysing patterns of induction in normal and these variant MELC lines suggests that the loss of proliferative capacity involves a complex multi-step process. Cells progress through an initial series of inducer-mediated changes which are characterized by a variety of metabolic alterations, but which are not associated with a commitment to terminal differentiation. Accumulation of factors determining commitment occurs after this inital period, generally beginning about 8 to 10 hours after onset of culture with inducer. Expression of the characteristics of terminal differentiation, including terminal cell division and the erythroid cells specific genes, e.g. globin genes (Chen *et al.*, 1982) can be detected by 12-15hrs.

EXPRESSION OF GLOBIN GENES

In the present review, we focus on investigations in our laboratory which have examined the effects of inducer on the expression of α and β globin genes during inducer-mediated MELC differentiation. Terminal erythroid cell differentiation of normal erythroid precursors requires the action of the erythropoietic hormone, erythropoietin (Marks and Rifkind, 1978). Viral transformed MELC appear to have become erythropoietin independent, and neither require the hormone for growth in culture, nor does the hormone induce them to express characteristics of terminal erythroid cell differentiation. On the other hand, a broad series of chemicals will induce differentiation of MELC, including the expression of α and β globin genes (Table 1).

In this paper, we specifically address two aspects of inducer-mediated MELC expression of α and β globin genes.

P.A. Marks *et al.*

TABLE 1
*Inducers of MELC Erythroid Differentiation**

Polar compounds:	Dimethylsulfoxide
	Hexamethylene bisacetamide
Fatty acids:	Butyric acid
DNA intercalators:	Actinomycin
Modified bases:	Azacytidine
Phosphodiesterase inhibitors:	Methylisoxanthine
Ion-flux agents:	Ouabain
Physical agents:	u.v., x-ray
Post-transcription-acting agents:	Haemin

*For detailed references see review (1).(Marks and Rifkind, 1978)

First, we have found that different inducers cause different patterns of expression of the α and β globin genes, during MELC differentiation, which appears due, in part, to the fact that inducers act at different levels of control of globin gene expression. Secondly, using various assays to evaluate chromatin structure, we have found that transcriptional activation of globin structural genes is associated with a complex set of changes in the configuration of globin gene chromatin (Sheffery *et al.*, 1982; 1983a and b; Hofer *et al.*, 1982). Certain patterns of chromatin structure have been established prior to the block in MELC erythropoiesis and these changes are stably propagated. These patterns, it is suggested, represent, at a molecular level, the developmental history of this transformed erythroid precursor. Other alterations in chromatin structure occur during the course of inducer-mediated MELC differentiation and the expression of the α and β globin genes. These changes, presumably, reflect in part molecular events characteristic of the final stages of differentiation of this lineage. Taken together, these findings suggest that the transition from a relatively inactive to an actively transcribed set of genes, using the globin genes as a model, appears to involve a complex process which is characterized, at least in part, by a series of alterations in chromatin configuration in the domain of these genes.

DIFFERENT EFFECTS OF INDUCERS ON EXPRESSION OF GLOBIN GENES IN MELC DIFFERENTIATION

MELC accumulate two types of haemoglobin, containing three species of globin polypeptides (α, β^{maj}, and β^{min}). Thus, inducer-mediated accumulation of haemoglobin may involve the coordinated expression of at least three different genes. All inducers of MELC (Table 1) can increase the accumulation of haemoglobin. It has been found that in uninduced MELC, there is a low but detectable level of Hb^{min} reflecting a low level of α and β^{min} globin gene expression in uninduced MELC (Nudel et al., 1977a). Polar-Planar compounds, such as HMBA and Me_2SO, induce the accumulation of two-fold or more Hb^{maj} than Hb^{min}. Butyric and propionic acids induce approximately equal amounts of Hb^{maj} and Hb^{min}. Haemin induces the accumulation of predominantly Hb^{min} (Nudel et al., 1977a; Curtis et al., 1980).

Studies of the rates of accumulation of α, β^{maj} and β^{min} globin mRNA show that these reflect closely the relative rates of accumulation of Hb^{maj} and Hb^{min} in MELC induced with the different agents studied, including Me_2SO, HMBA butyric acid and haemin (Nudel et al., 1977a). We have found differences in the kinetics of appearance as well as in the relative amounts of α and β globin mRNA, with different inducers. When MELC are cultured in the presence of HMBA, Me_2SO or butyric acid, accumulation of α globin mRNA can be detected in the cytoplasm by 12 to 16 h (Nudel et al., 1977a and b). Cytoplasmic accumulation of β globin mRNA sequences is not detected until about 8 h later, in the presence of these inducers. By 48 h there is an approximately ten-fold increase in the globin mRNA content of induced MELC. Haemin, by comparison, unlike the polar compounds (such as Me_2SO and HMBA) or the fatty acids (such as butyric acid), rapidly (by 6 h) and simultaneously initiates the accumulation of both α and β globin mRNA. Although the principal β-like mRNA induced by the polar inducers is β^{maj} mRNA, haemin initiates accumulation of β^{min} globin mRNA which is the principal β globin found in uninduced MECL.

INDUCER-MEDIATED EFFECTS ON GLOBIN GENE TRANSCRIPTION

The finding of differences in patterns of haemoglobins and globin mRNA accumulation in MELC induced with different agents led us to study the molecular level at which inducers affect control of gene expression. We turned first to investigate transcriptional control of the α_1 and β^{maj} globin genes. For these studies, we employed the technique of the nuclear chain elongation transcription assay (Hofer et al., 1982). We compared the effects of two inducers of MELC, namely, HMBA and

haemin.   Isolated nuclei, prepared from cells cultured with
one or the other of these agents, were incubated with ^{32}P-UTP
for five min.   RNA polymerase II-generated RNA molecules,
already associated with DNA templates, will be elongated with
^{32}P-UTP under these conditions and the level of radioactivity
associated with the gene-specific nascent RNA may be taken as
a measure of gene-specific transcriptional activity.

RNA was isolated from the nuclei and hybridized to a series
of double-stranded subclones prepared from the β^{maj} globin
gene and the α_1 globin gene (Sheffery *et al.*, 1983 ; Hofer *et
al.*, 1982.   For the β^{maj} globin gene domain, restriction
enzyme-generated fragments extending approximately 1.5 kb 5'
(upstream) to approximately 1.4 kb 3' (downstream) from the
structural gene were prepared.   Of these one fragment upstream and two fragments downstream did not contain sequences
corresponding to the structural portions of the β^{maj} globin
gene.   For the α_1 globin gene domain, restriction enzyme-
generated fragments extending approximately 2.3 kb up-stream
and 0.4 kb downstream from the structural gene were prepared.
Of these two fragments upstream and one fragment downstream
did not contain sequences corresponding to the structural sequences of the α_1 globin gene.   For the β^{maj} globin gene,
three fragments and for the α_1 globin gene, four fragments
contain structural sequences.

In the ^{32}P-labelled nuclear chain elongation transcript RNA
isolated from nuclei of MELC cultured with HMBA for 48 h, the
transcripts show a markedly increased hybridization to the
fragments of the α_1 globin gene and to the fragments of the
β globin gene which contain structural sequences compared with
comparable preparations from MELC cultured either without
inducer or with haemin.   Transcription of both the α_1 and β^{maj}
globin genes increases approximately 10 to 20-fold after 48 h
of culture with HMBA.   These findings suggest that the HMBA-
mediated increase in accumulation of α and β globin mRNA reflects, primarily, control of gene expression exercised at the
level of transcription.   By comparison, haemin appears to
effect an increase in globin mRNA accumulation without accel-
erating the rate of transcription (Profous-Juchelka *et al.*,
1983).   By implication, this means that haemin acts at a post-
transcriptional level, influencing the processing, transport
or stability of a low but constitutive level of transcript.
This mechanism appears consistent with the known effect of
haemin in augmenting the content of Hb^{min}, which is the principle haemoglobin, albeit at very low level, of uninduced MELC
(Nudel *et al.*, 1977a; Curtis *et al.*, 1980).

ALTERATIONS IN CHROMATIN STRUCTURE IN GLOBIN GENE DOMAINS

From the findings summarized above, it is clear that during
HMBA-induced MELC differentiation there is a 10 to 20-fold
increase in the rate of transcription of the α_1 and β^{maj} globin genes. Studies from a number of laboratories have established that alterations in DNA and chromatin structure are
associated with gene expression in differentiating cell systems (for reviews see Profous-Juchelka *et al.*, 1983; Weisbrod,
1982; Elgin, 1981; Ogo-Kemenes *et al.*, 1982). These include
changes in the patterns of DNA methylation (Felsenfeld and
McGhee, 1982; Doerfier, 1981), in binding of high mobility
group (MHG) proteins 14 and 17 (Weisbrod and Weintraub, 1979),
sensitivity ot chromatin to digestion by DNase I (Weintraub
and Groudine, 1976; Garel and Axel, 1976), and the appearance
of sites or regions that are hypersensitive to digestion by
DNase I, usually (but not invariably) found upstream of the
5' end of active (or potentially active) genes (Elgin, 1981;
Larsen and Weintraub, 1982).

Sites of S_1-nuclease sensitivity have recently been demonstrated to be associated with, but not necessarily identical to
sites of DNase I hypersensitivity (Sheffery *et al.*, 1983 ;
Larsen and Weintraub, 1982). McGee, Felsenfeld and co-workers
(McGhee *et al.*, 1981) have demonstrated that the DNase I hypersensitive region adjacent to the active chick β globin gene is
in a configuration suggesting the absence of normal nucleo-
somal structures and the presence of a stretch of protein-free
DNA.

Several features of DNA and chromatic configuration have
been examined in detail in our laboratory with respect to
changes in gene expression at the globin loci during induced
MELC differentiation (Sheffery *et al.*, 1982). Alterations in
chromatic structure in the domain of the α_1 and β^{maj} globin
structural genes have been evaluated by determination of:
1) the pattern of DNA methylation, 2) the sensitivity to
DNase I, 3) the pattern of chromatin sites hypersensitive to
DNase I digestion and 4) the pattern of chromatin sites sensitive to S_1 nuclease digestion. Certain patterns of chromatin
and DNA are found in uninduced MELC which fail to change upon
induction of terminal cell differentiation; these include the
pattern of DNA methylation about both the α_1 and β^{maj} genes,
and the general sensitivity of these genes to DNase I. On the
other hand, other changes occur during induction of differentiation; these include the development of DNase I hypersensitive sites and S_1 nuclease sensitive sites 5' to both the α_1
and β^{maj} genes.

Thus, certain changes in chromatin structure have already
occurred, presumably during the developmental history of the

erythroid lineage, and are stably propagated in the virus transformed, developmentally arrested, MELC. Additional changes in chromatin structure occur only when exposure to inducers initiates terminal differentiation.

DNA Methylation

The pattern of DNA methylation has been cited as a heritable molecular charactsristic which, at least in many instances, distinguishes expressed and unexpressed genes (Feisenfeld and McGhee, 1982; Doerfier, 1981). In general, relative hypo-methylation is associated with activation of transcription of a structural gene sequence; however, not all potential methyl-ation sites within a domain need be unmethylated and unique sites may well be critical for active transcription. For ex-ample, in the rabbit β globin domain, demethylation of some, but not all methylated sites correlates with gene activity (McGhee *et al.*, 1981). A small decrease in overall DNA methyl-ation has been described during induced differentiation of MELC (Weintraub *et al.*, 1981).

We examined the pattern of DNA methylation in the region of the β^{maj} and α_1 globin genes during HMBA-mediated MELC dif-ferentiation. Cytosine methylation in the nucleotide sequence, CCGG, was assayed by use of the methy-sensitive isoschizomer-pair of restriction enzymes, Msp I and Hpa II and other re-striction enzymes (Sheffery *et al.*, 1982). Compared to the nucleotide and methylation pattern in the chick (Weintraub *et al.*, 1981) there are relatively few potentially methylated sites in the MELC globin gene domains which can be assayed by these restriction enzymes.

Of the sites assayed and mapped near the β^{maj} globin gene, one site is fully methylated, one is partially methylated, and one is unmethylated in uninduced cells. Most sites (but not all) assayed near the α_1 globin genes are unmethylated in un-induced cells. No detectable change in the pattern of DNA methylation around either the α_1 or β^{maj} globin genes was ob-served during HMBA-mediated differentiation. It would appear that, within the limits of resolution of this assay, the pat-tern of globin methylation is established and stably propagated at a developmental stage in erythropoiesis prior to the stage represented by the MELC. This pattern is not required to change during subsequent transition to active globin expression.

DNase I Sensitivity

Previous studies of the accessibility of MELC chromatin diges-tion by DNase I, as assayed by liquid hybridization (Miller *et al.*, 1978), suggested that the globin gene-associated

chromatin of uninduced MELC is in an "active" configuration
relatively accessible to nuclease action, as compared to the
chromatin about other genes not expressed in erythroid cells.
We have examined, by the method of Southern, (1975), the
DNase I accessibility of α_1 and β^{maj} globin genes, in comparison with the sensitivity of another gene locus Igα, which
is not expressed in MELC. The β^{maj}- and α_1-globin genes are
distinctly more sensitive to digestion by DNase I than is the
Igα gene, uninduced and induced MELC.

Taken together, the observations on methylation pattern and
general DNase I sensitivity suggest that the α_1 and β^{maj} globin
gene domains of MELC, before their induction to full transcriptional activity, are in a differentiation-specific configuration compatible with and perhaps essential for the induction of globin gene expression.

DNase I Hypersensitivity Sites

We have obtained evidence for alterations in chromatin structure specifically associated with inducer-mediated activation
of globin gene transcription (Sheffery et al., 1982). During
HMBA-induced differentiation of MELC, specific sites, display-
ing a six- to ten-fold increase in DNase I sensitivity, appear
in chromatin regions near the 5' end of the α_1 and β^{maj} globin
genes. The DNase I hypersensitive site near the β^{maj} globin
gene maps to an approximately 200 bp region in the 5'-flanking
region of the gene. A DNase hypersensitive site is similarly
generated, during activation of globin gene expression, 5' to
the α_1 globin gene.

The changes in chromatin structure which are revealed by
nuclease probes during induced differentiation are more complex than the reconfiguration of sites at the 5' end of the
globin genes. Thus, there is a DNase I hypersensitivity site,
located within the second IVS of the β^{maj} gene, present in uninduced MELC (Sheffery et al., 1984). The nuclease sensitivity at this site decreases during HMBA-mediated MELC differentiation, and the new hypersensitivity site which lies 5' to
the β^{maj} cap site appears. This complex change in chromatin
configuration takes place in a coordinate fashion in inducer
sensitive DS19 cells prior to the initiation of globin gene
transcription.

The variant MELC line, R1, is resistant to HMBA induction
to terminal cell division and haemoglobin accumulation, but
exhibits other changes associated with inducer mediated terminal erythroid differentiation (Marks et al., 1983). In this
inducer-resistant variant the changes in chromatin configuration can be dissociated. In R1 cells HMBA mediates the disappearance of the hypersensitivity site located in IVS-2 but

fails to generate the new site, located 5' to the β^{maj} cap
site, and fails to initiate transcription at the β^{maj} gene
(Sheffery *et al.*, 1983b).

At the α_1 domain, there is also a complex pattern of chromatin reconfiguration that occurs during induced differentiation (Sheffery *et al.*, 1984). In uninduced MELC, overlapping
DNase and S_1 nuclease-sensitive sites are detected 5'
of the -globin gene cap site. During induction, the nuclease
sensitivity of these sites increases and new, non-overlapping
DNase I and S_1 sites develop, one approximately 300 base pairs
5' of the α_1 globin cap site, and the other mapping to a
region virtually coincident with the cap site itself. None
of these changes in nuclease sensitivity occur in the variant
R1 cells, suggesting that the changes in chromatin structure
5' to the cap site of both the β^{maj} and α_1 globin genes is a
prerequisite for inducer mediated activation of globin gene
transcription.

SUMMARY

This paper summarizes evidence that the transition from relatively inactive to actively expressed globin genes associated
with HMBA-induced MELC differentiation involves a complex
series of alterations in the chromatin structure of the genes.
We suggest that these virus-transformed cells, CFU-e like
erythroid precursors, have globin chromatin structure, characterized at least in part, by a particular DNA methylation pattern and a generally increased level of DNase sensitivity
which reflects the cells' developmental progression in the
erythroid lineage to a stage of potential globin gene transcription. In this model, these features of chromatin structure
of the globin genes may be associated with the restriction in
developmental potential characteristic of progression in the
haemopoietic lineage to a CFUe-like stage of erythropoiesis,
at which the transfromed MELC appear to be blocked. These
changes in chromatin structure are stably propagated in MELC
and constitute, as it were, the molecular phenotype of this
developmental stage.

The major increase in globin gene transcription which is
associated with HMBA-mediated terminal differentiation of
MELC, is accompanied by further changes in chromatin structure,
as indicated, in part, by the appearance of DNase I hypersensitive and S_1 nuclease sensitive sites 5' to both the α_1
and βmaj globin genes. Taken together these observations
suggest that a multi-step alteration in chromatin structure
is associated with the developmental history of erythroid
cells and with the increased globin gene transcription which
occurs in the expression of terminal erythroid differentiation.

ACKNOWLEDGEMENTS

The studies summarized in this review performed in the laboratories of the authors were supported, in part, by grants from
the National Cancer Institute (PO1 CA-31768 and CA-08748) and
the Bristol-Myers Cancer Research Program.

REFERENCES

Boyer, S.H., Wuu, K.D., Noyes, A.M., Young, R., Scher, W.,
    Friend, C., Preisler, H. and Bank, A. (1972). *Blood* 40,
    823-835.
Chen, Z.X., Banks, J., Rifkind, R.A. and Marks, P.A. (1982).
    Proc. Natl. Acad. Sci. USA 79, 471-475.
Curtis, P., Finnigan, A.C. and Robera, G. (1980). *J. Biol.
    Chem.* 255, 8971-8974.
Doerfler, W. (1981). *J. Gen. Virol.* 57, 1-20.
Eisen, H., Nasi, S., Georopulos, C.P., Arndt-Jovin, D. and
    Ostertag, W. (1977). *Cell* 10, 680-695.
Eisen, H., Keppel-Bellivet, F., Georgopoulos, C.P., Sassa, S.,
    Granick, J., Pragnell, I. and Astertog, W. (1978). *In*
    "Cold Spring Harbor Conferences on Cell Proliferation"
    (Eds. Clarkson, Marks and Till) 5, 277-294.
Elgin, S.C.R. (1981). *Cell* 27, 413-415.
Felsenfeld, G. and McGhee, J. (1982). *Nature* 296, 602-603.
Fibach, E., Reuben, R.C., Rifkind, R.A. and Marks, P.A. (1977).
    Cancer Res. 37, 440-444.
Friend, C., Scher, W., Holland, J.G. and Sato, T. (1971).
    Proc. Natl. Acad. Sci. USA 68, 378-82.
Garel, A. and Axel, R. (1976). *Proc. Natl. Acad. Sci. USA*
    73, 3966-3970.
Gusella, J., Geller, R., Clarke, B., Weeks, V. and Housman, D.
    (1976). *Cell* 9, 221-229.
Hofer, E., Hofer-Warbinek, R. and Darnell, J.E. (1982). *J. Cell*
    29, 887-893.
Keppel, F., Allet, B. and Eisen, H. (1977). *Proc. Natl. Acad.
    Sci. USA* 74, 653-656.
Larsen, A. and Weintraub, H. (1982). *Cell* 29, 609-622.
Leder, A. and Leder, P. (1975). *Cell* 5, 319-322.
Levenson, R. and Housman, D. (1981). *Cell* 25, 5-6.
Levenson, R., Kerner, J. and Housman, D. (1979). *Cell* 18,
    1073-1078.
McGhee, J.D., Wood, W.I., Dolan, M., Engel, J.D. and Felsenfeld,
    G. (1981). *Cell* 27, 45-55.
Marks, P.A. and Rifkind, R.A. (1978). *Ann. Rev. Biochem.* 47,
    419-448.
Marks, P.A., Rifkind, R.A., Bank, A., Terada, Md., Gambari, R.,
    Ribach, E., Maniatis, G. and Reuben, R.C. (1979). *In*

"Cellular and Molecular Regulation of Hemoglobin Switching" (Eds. G. Stamatoyannopolulos and A.W. Neinhuis), pp.437-455. Grune and Stratton, New York.

Marks, P.A., Chen, Z.X., Banks, J. and Rifkind, R.A. (1983). *Proc. Natl. Acad. Sci.* 80, 2281-2284.

Miller, D.M., Turner, P., Nienhuis, A.W., Axelrod, D.E. and Gopalakrishman, T.V. (1978). *Cell* 14, 511-524.

Nudel, U., Salmon, J., Fibach, E., Terada, M., Rofkind, R.A., Marks, P.A. and Bank, A. (1977a). *Cell* 12, 463-469.

Nudel, U., Salmon, J.D., Terada, M., Bank, A., Rifkind, R.A. and Marks, P.A. (1977b). *Proc. Natl. Acad. Sci. USA* 74, 1100-1104.

Ogo-Kemenes, T., Horz, W. and Zachau, H.G. (1982). *Ann. Rev. Biochem.* 51, 89-121.

Ohta, Y., Tanaka, M., Terada, M., Miller, O.J., Bank, A., Marks, P.A. and Rifkind, R.A. (1976). *Proc. Natl. Acad. Sci. USA* 73, 1232-1236.

Ostertag, W., Melderis, H., Steinheider, G., Kluge, N. and Dube, S. (1972). *Nature (London) New Biol.* 239, 231-234.

Pragnell, I.B., Arudt-Jovin, D.J., Jovin, T.M., Fogg, B. and Astertog, W. (1980). *Exper. Cell Res.* 125, 459-470.

Profous-Juchelka, H.R., Reuben, R.C., Marks, P.A. and Rifkind, R.A. (1983). *Mol. and Cell Biol.* Vol. 3, 2, 229-232.

Reuben, R.C., Wife, R.L., Breslow, R., Rifkind, R.A. and Marks, P.A. (1976). *Proc. Natl. Acad. Sci. USA* 73, 862-866.

Ross, J., Ikawa, Y. and Leder, P. (1972). *Proc. Natl. Acad. Sci. USA* 69, 3620-3623.

Sassa, S. (1976). *J. Exp. Med.* 143, 305-315.

Sheffery, M., Rifkind, R.A. and Marks, P.A. (1982). *Proc. Natl. Acad. Sci. USA* 79, 1180-1184.

Sheffery, M., Rifkind, R.A. and Marks, P.A. (1983). *Proc. Natl. Acad. Sci. USA* 80, 3349-3353.

Sheffery, M., Rifkind, R.A. and Marks, P.A. (1984). *J. Mol. Biol.* 172, 417-436.

Southern, E.M. (1975). *J. Mol. Biol.* 98, 503-517.

Weintraub, H., Larsen, A. and Groudine, M. (1981). *Cell* 24, 333-344.

Weintraub, H. and Groudine, M. (1976). *Science* 193, 848-856.

Weisbrod, S. (1982). *Nature* 297, 289-295.

Weisbrod, S. and Weintraub, H. (1979). *Proc. Natl. Acad. Sci. USA* 76, 630-634.

THE FUNCTION OF SIGNAL RECOGNITION PARTICLE (SRP) AND SRP-RECEPTOR IN THE PROCESS OF PROTEIN TRANSLOCATION ACROSS THE ENDOPLASMIC RETICULUM MEMBRANE

P. Walter, R. Gilmore* and G. Blobel*

*Department of Biochemistry and Biophysics,
University of California San Francisco, California 94143, USA*

*The Rockefeller University New York, New York 10021, USA

An important aspect of the biosynthesis of proteins is their intracellular topology (Blobel, 1980). Many proteins spend their entire lives in the same compartment in which they are synthesized; others have to cross the hydrophobic barrier of distinct cellular membranes in order to reach the intra-cellular compartment or extracellular site where they exert their function. Numerous membrane proteins have to be asymmetrically integrated into distinct cellular membranes. For many proteins this requires partial translocation, i.e. the selective transfer of distinct hydrophilic domains of their polypeptide chain across specific membranes.

Although there are several translocation competent intra-cellular membrane systems in a eukaryotic cell (Blobel, 1980), we will focus here only on the translocation system of the rough endoplasmic reticulum (RER), where secretory (Palade, 1975) and lysosomal (Erickson *et al.*, 1981) proteins are co-translationally translocated across and certain membrane proteins (Lingappa *et al.*, 1978) are co-translationally integrated into the membrane. To explain how, during their biosynthesis, these proteins are targeted to and translocated across the RER, the "Signal Hypothesis" was formulated (Blobel and Dobberstein, 1975a). In brief, it was postulated that the nascent polypeptide, as it emerges from the ribosome, expresses as part of its amino acid sequence, the information (the "Signal Sequence") which causes the ribosome involved to attach to the membrane of the RER. There, RER-specific integral membrane

proteins recognize the signal sequence and, in response, form
a hydrophilic "pore" which allows the nascent chain to be vec-
torially translocated across the membrane. Upon termination
of protein synthesis, the ribosome detaches from the membrane
and the permeability barrier is restored.

Until recently, the proposed recognition and translocation
machinery (Blobel, 1980; Blobel and Dobberstein, 1975a; Blobel
and Sabatini, 1971; Milstein *et al.*, 1972) remained largely
undefined and, as a consequence, several hypotheses were put
forward suggesting that targeting and translocation take place
without mediation by other proteins (Bretscher, 1973; von
Heijne and Blomberg, 1979; Wickner, 1979; Garnier *et al.*,
1980; Engelman and Steitz, 1981). Only after the development
of *in vitro* translocation systems (Blobel and Dobberstein,
1975b; Szczesna and Boime, 1975) that were able to reproduce
translocation of nascent secretory proteins across the RER-
membrane (isolated in the form of closed microsomal vesicles)
with apparent fidelity, did a detailed biochemical analysis
of this process become feasible. So far, two components have
been purified from dog pancreas and shown to be required in
this translocation process.

One of these is the so-called Signal Recognition Particle
(SRP), an 11S ribonucleoprotein (RNP) (Walter and Blobel,
1982). SRP consists of six non-identical polypeptide chains
(72, 68, 54, 19, 14 and 9 kd) (Walter and Blobel, 1980) and
one molecule of 7S RNA (Walter and Blobel, 1982). Both RNA
and protein are required for SRP's activity (Walter and Blobel,
1982). In dog pancreas at physiological salt concentration
(150 mM potassium ions) the bulk of the SRP appears to be
equally distributed between a RER-bound state and a free ribo-
some/polysome-associated form (Walter and Blobel, 1983).

The RNA in SRP has been identified by sequence analysis
(Walter and Blobel, 1982b) to be identical to the small cytoplasmic 7SL RNA (Ullu *et al.*, 1982d) (alternatively known as
7S scRNA (Walker *et al.*, 1974) and ScL RNA (Zieve and Penman,
1976). 7SL was first described as a component of some oncorna-
viruses (Bishop *et al.*, 1970), but later shown to be a constitutive component of all uninfected cells (Erickson *et al.*,
1973). It was variously localized (Walker *et al.*, 1975;
Zieve and Penman, 1976; Gunning *et al.*, 1981) in ribosomal,
microsomal, as well as nuclear cell fractions (Reddy *et al.*,
1981). It is a relatively stable RNA (with a slow turnover
rate) which has been highly conserved through evolution
(Walker *et al.*, 1974; Erikson *et al.*, 1973; Reddy *et al.*,
1981). Recently, it was sequenced both by using a cDNA clone
of the human RNA (Ullu *et al.*, 1982a and b) and by direct RNA
sequencing of the rat RNA (Li *et al.*, 1982). The sequences
obtained were essentially identical (Walter and Blobel, 1982)

and confirmed a previous observation (Weiner, 1980) that long
stretches of 7SL RNA are homologous to the Alu family DNA sequences. Thus, the about 300 nucleotide long 7SL RNA was
shown to have about 80% homology to the Alu consensus sequence
(Deininger *et al.*, 1981) for about 100 nucleotides at its 5'
end and 50 nucleotides at its 3' end (Ullu *et al.*, 1982a; Li
et al., 1982). However, the core-portion of 7SL RNA (about
150 nucleotides) showed no homology to Alu DNA, and is comple-
mentary to a new family of repeated DNA (but repeated at a
lower frequency than Alu DNA) in the genome (Ullu *et al.*,
1982a). Little is known about the function of 7SL-RNA or the
significance of Alu-like sequences in SRP. However, it could
be shown that dissociated SRP proteins behave as inactive
monomers or dimers and require 7SL-RNA to recombine into active 11S SRP (Walter and Blobel, 1983a). Thus, at least one
function of 7SL-RNA in SRP is a structural one, namely to
provide a matrix for the coordinated assembly of the particle.
   The second isolated component of the protein translocation
machinery, the SRP-receptor (Gilmore *et al.*, 1982a) (also
termed "Docking Protein" (Meyer *et al.*, 1982a) is a protein
of 72 kd (Gilmore *et al.*, 1982a; Meyer *et al.*, 1982b) that
has been purified from detergent-solubilized microsomal membranes by affinity chromatography on SRP-Sepharose (Gilmore
et al., 1982a). The SRP-receptor is an integral membrane protein, restricted in its subcellular distribution to the membrane system of the RER. It consists of a large cytoplasmic
domain of 60 kd (Meyer and Dobberstein, 1980a) that can be
severed from the membrane by treatment with a variety of
proteases and can be added to the proteolysed membranes to
reconstitute activity (Gilmore *et al.*, 1982b; Walter *et al.*,
1979; Meyer and Dobberstein, 1980b).
   The function of these components (SRP and SRP receptor) in
the protein translocation process was deduced using *in vitro*
assembled translating polysomes which were programmed with
mRNA coding for secretory proteins. Thus, it became possible
to follow directly the fate of a nascent secretory protein
and thereby to analyse the discrete steps of its recognition
and its subsequent translocation across the membrane of microsomal vesicles.
   The data accumulated so far are discussed in the model depicted in Fig. 1 (taken from Walter and Blobel, 1981). It
was shown (Meyer *et al.*, 1982a; Walter *et al.*, 1981; Walter
and Blobel, 1983a) that free (soluble) SRP existed in equilibrium with a membrane-bound form (interacting with the SRP
receptor) (Fig. 1A), as well as with a ribosome-bound form
(Fig. 1B). Upon translation of an mRNA specifically coding
for a signal sequence that is addressed to the RER translocation system (Fig. 1C), there was an enhancement of the

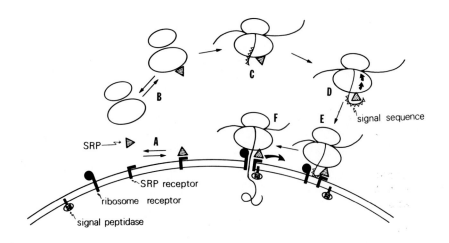

FIG. 1   (From Walter and Blobel, 1981)

apparent affinity of SRP for the translating ribosome of
several orders of magnitude (Fig. 1D) (Walter *et al.*, 1981).
Thus, SRP was found to *recognize* the signal sequence of nascent
secretory (Walter *et al.*, 1981; Stoffel *et al.*, 1981; Mueller
et al., 1982), lysosomal (Erikson *et al.*, 1983), and membrane
(Anderson *et al.*, 1982) proteins. It is not known what the
actual recognizable consensus feature is, since signal sequences lack primary sequence homology (Blobel *et al.*, 1979).
    Interestingly, concomitant with this increase in binding
affinity, SRP *specifically arrested* the elongation of the
initiated polypeptide chain (just after the signal peptide had
emerged from the ribosome) (Fig. 1D), and thereby prevented
the completion of the pre-secretory protein (Meyer *et al.*,
1982a; Walter and Blobel, 1981; Walker *et al.*, 1981). Upon
interaction of these arrested ribisomes with the SRP receptor
on the microsomal membrane, this elongation arrest was released
(Meyer *et al.*, 1982a; Gilmore *et al.*, 1982b; Walter and Blobel,
1981) and the nascent chain was translocated across (Walter
and Blobel, 1981) or, as in the case of integral membrane
proteins, integrated into (Anderson *et al.*, 1982) the lipid
bilayer (Fig. 1E).
    The mechanism by which SRP interacts with the ribosome and
signal sequences to cause elongation arrest and how SRP receptor acts to release this arrest is unknown. However, it
has been speculated (Walter and Blobel, 1981) that it might
be physiologically important to prevent the complete synthesis
of secretory and lysosomal proteins in the cytoplasm. SRP-
mediated elongation arrest could also be of important regu-

latory significance. Modulation of the arrest releasing
activity either by other as yet unidentified components or by
direct modification of SRP and/or the SRP receptor could provide the cell with an on-off switch for translocation-coupled
protein synthesis and thereby provide a mechanism for a fast
and regulatable response to a variety of physiological stimuli.

It was estimated (Walter and Blobel, 1980; Gilmore
1982a) that the stoichiometry of bound ribosomes to SRP receptor to SRP is about 25:5:1 in the microsome fraction. Thus,
the content of both SRP and SRP receptor is less than that of
bound ribosomes. This suggested (Walter and Blobel, 1981)
that the ribosome-SRP-SRP receptor interaction might be a
transient one, merely targeting the SRP-arrested ribosome to
a specific, translocation competent site on the RER membrane.
This assumption has been recently confirmed (Gilmore and
Blobel, 1983). It was possible to demonstrate that when purified and labelled SRP-receptor in detergent solution was used
to release the elongation arrest of polysomes, both SRP and
SRP-receptor dissociated from the translating ribosomes and
no longer bound with detectable affinity. It follows that
once targeting has occurred, the ribosome-SRP-SRP receptor
interaction is replaced (Fig. 1F) by a direct interaction of
the ribosomes with other integral membrane proteins (here indicated as a putative ribosome receptor), thus freeing SRP
and SRP receptor to be recycled. Two integral membrane proteins (ribophorin I and II) which might function as ribosome
receptors have been described by Kreibich, Sabatini and co-
workers (Kreibich *et al.*, 1978a and b; Marcantonio *et al.*,
1982) and appear to be involved in ribosome binding to the
RER. However, their direct involvement in protein translocation has not yet been demonstrated and has been questioned
by other investigators (Bielinska *et al.*, 1979). Thus, at
present there is no direct proof that other integral membrane
proteins besides the SRP receptor are required for protein
translocation across the RER. It should also be noted that
essentially no experimental data on the mechanism of the
actual transmembrane movement of the nascent chain are currently available. The depicted "pore" in the membrane in Fig. 1
should therefore presently be interpreted as a local environment in the lipid bilayer that will allow the passage of the
polypeptide chain.

Finally, it should be noted that both SRP (Mueller *et al.*,
1982) and 7SL RNA (Walker *et al.*, 1974; Erikson *et al.*, 1973;
Reddy *et al.*, 1981)) and the mode of co-translational protein
translocation (Blobel, 1980; Chang *et al.*, 1979) appear to be
highly conserved through evolution. Thus, it was recently
possible to demonstrate (Mueller *et al.*, 1982) that the signal
sequence of a nascent prokaryotic secretory protein (beta-

lactamase), which was synthesized on plant ribosomes (wheat germ), was correctly recognized by mammalian SRP (canine), i.e. elongation was arrested and translocation across mammalian membranes was SRP dependent. Another line of evidence for the highly conserved nature of SRP is derived from reconstitution experiments of SRP itself (Walter and Blobel, 1983a). We were able to prepare "chimeric SRPs" consisting of mammalian proteins and either amphibian or insect 7SL-RNA and to show that these particles work with fidelity in *in vitro* assays. SRP therefore appears to be an integral and indispensable component of the protein synthesis machinery of living cells assuring the correct topogenesis (Blobel, 1980) (the process by which newly synthesized proteins are transported to their correct subcellular localizations) of a specific subset of proteins. Considering its structural features and its intimate (although most likely transient) functional association with ribosomes, it could almost be regarded as a "third ribosomal subunit" functioning as the adapter between the cytoplasmic translation and the membrane-bound translocation machinery.

REFERENCES

Anderson, D.J., Walter, P. and Blobel, G. (1982). *J. Cell Biol.* 93, 501.
Bielinska, M., Rogers, G., Rucinsky, T. and Boime, I. (1979). *Proc. Natl. Acad. Sci. USA* 76, 6152.
Bishop, J.M., Levinson, W., Sullivan, D., Farrshien, L., Quintrell, N. and Jackson, J. (1970). *Virology* 42, 927.
Blobel, G. (1980). *Proc. Natl. Acad. Sci. USA* 77, 1496.
Blobel, G. and Dobberstein, B. (1975a). *J. Cell Biol.* 67, 835.
Blobel, G. and Dobberstein, B. (1975b). *J. Cell Biol.* 67, 852.
Blobel, G. and Sabatini, D.D. (1971). *Biomembranes* (Ed. L.A. Manson), Vol.2, pp.193-195. Plenum Press, New York.
Blobel, G., Walter, P., Chang, C.N., Goldman, B.M., Erickson, A.H. and Lingappa, V.R. (1979). *Soc. Exp. Biol. Symp.* (Eds. C.R. Hopkins and C.J. Duncan). Vol.33, pp.9-36. Cambridge University Press, Cambridge.
Bretscher, M.S. (1973). *Science* 181, 622.
Chang, C.N., Model, P. and Blobel, G. (1979). *Proc. Natl. Acad. Sci. USA* 76, 1251.
Deininger, P.L., Jolly, D.J., Rubin, C.M., Friedmann, T. and Schmid, J. (1981). *J. Mol. Biol.* 151, 17.
Engelman, D.M. and Steitz, T.A. (1981). *Cell* 23, 411.
Erikson, E., Erikson, R.L., Henry, B. and Pace, N.R. (1973). *Virology* 53, 40.
Erickson, A.H., Conner, G. and Blobel, G. (1981). *J. Biol. Chem.* 256, 11224.
Erickson, A.H., Walter, P. and Blobel, G. (1983). *Biochem. Biophys. Res. Comm.* 115, 275.

Garnier, J., Gaye, P., Mercier, J.C. and Robson, B. (1980).
  Biochimie 62, 231.
Gilmore, R. and Blobel, G. (1983). *Cell* 35, 677.
Gilmore, R., Walter, P. and Blobel, G. (1982a). *J. Cell Biol.*
  95, 470.
Gilmore, R., Blobel, G. and Walter, P. (1982b). *J. Cell. Biol.*
  95, 463.
Gunning, P.W., Beguin, P., Shooter, E.M., Austin, L. and
  Jeffrey, L. (1981). *J. Biol. Chem.* 256, 6670.
Kreibich, G., Ulrich, B.L. and Sabatini, D.D. (1978a). *J.*
  Cell Biol. 77, 464.
Kreibich, G., Freienstein, C.M., Pereyra, B.N., Ulrich, B.L.
  and Sabatini, D.D. (1978b). *J. Cell Biol.* 77, 488.
Li, W.Y., Reddy, R., Henning, D., Epstein, P. and Bush, H.
  (1982). *J. Biol. Chem.* 257, 5136.
Lingappa, V.R., Katz, F.N., Lodish, H.F. and Blobel, G. (1978).
  J. Biol. Chem. 253, 8667.
Marcantonio, E.E., Grebenan, R.C., Sabatini, D.D. and Kreibich,
  G. (1982). *Eur. J. Biochem.* 124, 217.
Meyer, D.I. and Dobberstein, B. (1980a). *J. Cell Biol.* 87,
  503.
Meyer, D.I. and Dobberstein, B. (1980b). *J. Cell Biol.* 87,
  498.
Meyer, D.I., Krause, E. and Dobberstein, B. (1982a). *Nature*
  (London) 297, 647.
Meyer, D.I., Louvard, D. and Dobberstein, B. (1982b). *J. Cell*
  Biol. 92, 579.
Milstein, C., Brownlee, G.G., Harrison, T.M. and Mathews, M.B.
  (1972). *Nature* 239, 117.
Mueller, M., Ibrahimi, I., Chang, C.N., Walter, P. and Blobel,
  G. (1982). *J. Biol. Chem.* 257, 11860.
Palade, G. (1975). *Science* 189, 347.
Reddy, R., Li, W.Y., Henning, D., Choi, Y.C., Nohga, K. and
  Bush, H. (1981). *J. Biol. Chem.* 256, 8452.
Stoffel, W., Blobel, G. and Walter, P. (1981). *Eur. J. Biochem.*
  120, 519.
Szczesna, E. and Boime, I. (1975). *Proc. Natl. Acad. Sci. USA*
  73, 1179.
Ullu, E., Murphy, S. and Melli, M. (1982a). *Cell* 29, 195.
Ullu, E. and Melli, M. (1982b). *Nuc. Acid Res.* 10, 2209.
von Heijne, C. and Blomberg, C. (1979). *Eur. J. Biochem.* 97,
  175.
Walker, T.A., Pace, N.R., Erikson, R.L., Erikson, E. and Behr,
  F. (1974). *Proc. Natl. Acad. Sci. USA* 71, 3390.
Walter, P. and Blobel, G. (1980). *Proc. Natl. Acad. Sci. USA*
  77, 7112.
Walter, P. and Blobel, G. (1981). *J. Cell Biol.* 91, 557.

Walter, P. and Blobel, G. (1982). *Nature (London)* 299, 691.

Walter, P. and Blobel, G. (1983a). *Cell* 34, 525.

Walter, P. and Blobel, G. (1983b). *J. Cell Biol.* 97, 1693.

Walter, P., Jackson, R.C., Marcus, M.M., Lingappa, V.R. and Blobel, G. (1979). *Proc. Natl. Acad. Sci. USA* 76, 1795.

Walter, P., Ibrahimi, I. and Blobel. G. (1981). *J. Cell Biol.* 91, 545.

Weiner, A. (1980). *Cell* 22, 209.

Wickner, W. (1979). *Annu. Rev. Biochem.* 48, 23.

Zieve, G. and Penman, S. (1976). *Cell* 8, 19.

INTESTINAL MICROFLORA AND CARCINOGENESIS

B.E. Gustafsson

*Department of Germfree Research,
Karolinska institutet, Stockholm, Sweden*

INTRODUCTION

Many investigators still have some difficulties when transfering results obtained in microorganisms by methods used within the field of molecular biology to those conditions in more complex cell systems as in higher organisms and in our own bodies.

The purpose of this paper is to try to demonstrate that the intestinal microflora has some properties which might fill this gap. When dealing with this entity, the medical profession has for obvious reasons been interested mostly in the pathogens. We have a tendency to forget that only one out of a thousand strains of microorganisms is a pathogen. Microorganisms in the intestines form an organ-like structure which in numbers and different strains infers that it is one of the largest entities of the body, with a weight close to that of the kidneys. Many of the normal functions that we register in the body are the results of activities of the normal microflora rather than of our own cells.

Many cancer disorders, as those in the intestines, pancreas and kidneys, have been related to diet. Other types of cancers discussed in this regard have been those of the breast, endometrium, ovaries, and the prostate.

On the other hand, Aries *et al.* (1969), proposed that some of the cancers in the intestinal tract were due to the action by intestinal bacteria on substrates, which by themselves were not carcinogenic. Evidence for such a mechanism was already presented in 1966 (Laqueur, 1964; Spatz *et al.*, 1966; Laqueur *et al.*, 1967) in the now classic investigation by Laqueur and collaborators. They demonstrated that the alkaloid cycasin,

THEORIES AND MODELS
IN CELLULAR TRANSFORMATION

which produces tumours in the intestinal tract when introduced
in the diet of conventional rats, was without such effect in
germfree rats.

Recent findings have led to the conclusion that many of the
classic interactions between carcinogens and body cells and
tissues have to be reinvestigated, with the question raised
whether microorganisms in the normal microbial flora are mediators in this respect.

From a principal point of view, an interception between
external factors and the body cells *per se* by the endogenous
microflora might be discussed against the following background:

1. Microorganisms may produce carcinogens from inactive compounds synthesized by the host. An example of this possibility would be the bile acids.
2. The effect of a known carcinogen could be brought about by
   metabolism by the microflora, which from a primarily in-
   nocuous compound in the diet produces active carcinogen.
   The already mentioned cycasin is a good example of this
   type of metabolic activation of a carcinogen.

INTESTINAL MICROFLORA - GENERAL PROBLEMS

Both the numbers of cells and the quantity of the microbial
flora in the intestines are rather astonishing. Considering
that the weight is about 1000 g in man, it is closer to that
of our large organs, the kidneys or the brain. The number of
cells being about 10^{13-14} per g (Luckey, 1977) means that there
are more living entities in the flora than there are cells in
our whole body. The number of different strains composing the
flora are estimated to be more than 500, some of which are
difficult or impossible to maintain in the laboratory due to
their nutritive requirements. The obligate anaerobes constitute 95% of the total number of bacteria (Finegold, 1970).
The dominant flora consists of some relatively unknown and
hard to isolate microorganisms. The original isolation is
also difficult because many of them are killed by rather short
exposure to ambient oxygen. Similar facts have been known for
many years concerning the gastric flora of ruminants.

The fate of the bacteria in the intestinal flora has to be
considered when the numbers, different strains, and interactions are evaluated. In a recent paper from our laboratory
(Midtvedt and Gustafsson, 1981) the possible digestion of mem-
bers of the microflora was investigated by feeding germfree
animals with killed suspensions of large numbers of bacteria
and following their appearance in the faeces. All Gram-
negative strains and certain strains of *Clostridia* were digested, most Gram-positive strains were not. Such differences

in digestibility could have both immunological and nutritional implications.

Another important feature of the intestinal flora is the formation of plaque-like structures on the epithelial surfaces. This bacterial film also extends down into the Lieberkühn's crypts (Gustafsson and Maunsbach, 1971), where almost pure strains are established in contrast to the great variety in the lumen. This again raises the question of the conditions in these crypts. The redox potential in a crypt within only fractions of microns from the epithelial cells is presumably quite low, about -300 mV.

The stability of this micro-environment has been demonstrated to us recently. We compared the contents of Lieberkühn's crypts in conventional rats of our strain of the 46th inbred generation in 1982 with the same of the 26th generation in 1969 as published in 1971 (Gustafsson and Maunsbach, 1971). A striking similarity is observed in the size and general morphology of the bacteria in the Lieberkühn's crypts in these animals investigated with a difference in time of more than ten years (Figs. 1 and 2).

The present concept of the intestinal bacterial flora is quite different from the earlier one, both from a morphological and physiological point of view. The flora, weighing about 1 kg, and thus equivalent to the larger organs of the body, is constructed as a long tube of densely packed bacteria anchored with villi-like extensions penetrating into the epithelial crypts. A portion of the intestinal flora and the contents are transported inside this tube of densely packed microorganisms, which seem to be very stable as far as composition and function are concerned.

GERM-FREE ANIMALS

A direct method for the study of the physiological and other properties of the normal microflora is the production and maintenance of germ-free animals. These were the principal subjects of our investigations in the past (Gustafsson, 1948; Reyniers *et al.*, 1949). The future will see greater use of germ-free animals produced by our standard methods, but also of animals contaminated with antibiotics.

A great number of characteristics of germ-free animals (enlarged caeca, etc.) have been recognized (Table 1). Many investigators initially thought anomalies could be easily corrected by contaminating the germ-free animals with well known inhabitants of the normal flora, such as strains of *E. coli*, *Lactobacilli* etc.

Although quite a few of the microorganisms necessary for the normal metabolism have been isolated, the situation in the

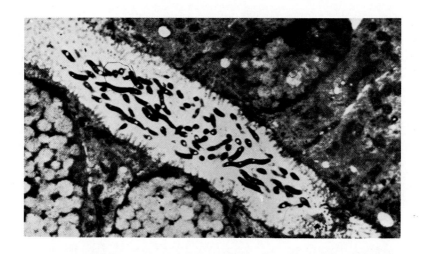

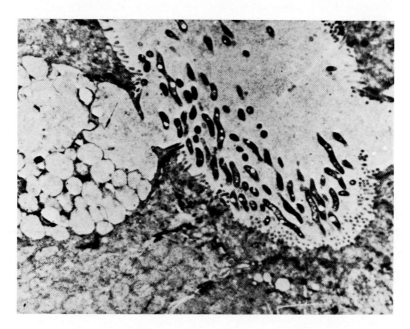

FIG. 1. *(Top) Crypt from a caecum of a conventional rat with only one morphological type of bacterium. The section was made in 1969 from a rat of the 26th generation of an inbred rat strain (AGUS).*

FIG. 2 *(Bottom) Crypt from the same site as Fig. 1 from a rat of the 46th generation in 1982 of the same rat strain as in Fig. 1. The preparation was thus made 13 years later than that in Fig. 1. Similarities with the bacteria in Fig. 1 are evident. Magnifications in both sections x 6400.*

TABLE 1

Characteristics of germ-free animals

A. Reticulo-endothelial system	1. Blood	- Immunoglobulin content low
	2. Lymphnodes	- Weight $\frac{1}{2}$ normal - No reaction centres - Few plasma cells
	3. Mucous membranes	- Few lymphoid cells
B. Intestinal tract	1. Intestines	- Redox potential reverted - Passage time increased - High faecal levels of trypsin and elastase - Mucin excreted in large, non-degraded amounts - Caecum enlarged with decreased motility - Lieberkühn's crypts widened
	2. Liver	- Higher activity of micro-somal hydroxylating enzyme systems - Stercobilin not formed
C. Steroids	1. Cholesterol	- Coprostanol not formed
	2. Bile acids	- No deconjugation - No 7α-dehydroxylation - Turnover $\frac{1}{2}$ of normal
	3. Steroid hormones	- No deconjugation - No 16α- or 21-dehydroxylation - Turnover $\frac{1}{2}$ of normal - Mineral metabolism altered

gut flora is far more complex than anticipated and is still not well understood. Many of the organisms which are able to correct symptoms in germ-free animals are anaerobic, very sensitive to ambient oxygen and fastidious in their growth requirements. They have, therefore, been difficult to isolate.

At this point, it is important to state that almost all of the symptoms or aberrations observed in germ-free animals can be produced in animals and man by the administration of relatively small doses of antibiotics for a few days, and that these symptoms might prevail for weeks and months after the administration has been stopped (Gustafsson and Norin, 1977; Gustafsson *et al.*, 1977). Also small amounts (i.e. 1/100 of the therapeutic dose) cause long term alterations of the function of the intestinal flora. This observation closes the gap between symptoms in germ-free animals and conditions seen in antibiotic treated patients.

Germ-free animals are presently used in a wide variety of studies, ranging from basic problems in physiology, metabolism, nutrition, immunobiology and microecology. These animals and the corresponding techniques are also used to study problems related to the metabolism and action of carcinogens.

CARCINOGENESIS

Studies in experimental animals have implicated the intestinal microflora in the aetiology of cancer through a number of mechanisms. These include:

1. Production of carcinogens, promotors and mutagens, as from bile acid metabolism, from amino acid metabolism, from azo dye metabolism and even from certain drugs. A much discussed possibility is formation of N-nitroso compounds from nitrites and amino compounds.
2. Release of carcinogenic aglycones from inactive conjugates.
3. Activation (promotion) and inactivation of carcinogens.
4. Modification of host defence mechanisms.

SPONTANEOUS TUMOURS IN GERM-FREE ANIMALS

Aging germ-free animals develop tumours with almost the same distribution as in control rats with a normal intestinal flora. Thus, Pollard and Luckert (1979) reported that liver tumours ranging from benign nodules to carcinomas developed spontaneously in 87% of 132 germ-free Wistar rats. In addition, the rats developed a high incidence of benign adenomas of endocrine glands and the breast. In our own colonies of old rats, both germ-free and conventional rats develop slow growing mammary adenofibromas and adenocarcinomas at ages of more than one year. Both groups have a high incidence of tumours in endocrine organs at ages higher than one year. Strains of germ-free mice in our laboratory have been found to have a very low incidence of tumours.

Although interesting observations have been made on the occurrence of spontaneous tumours in selected groups of aging germ-free animals, studies with systematic observations of larger numbers of animals during their entire life span are needed.

BILE ACID METABOLISM

Experimental animal evidence indicates that some secondary bile acids produced by the intestinal microflora might act as tumour promoting factors in the colon (Narisawa et al., 1974; Reddy et al., 1976; 1977). In vitro, lithocholic acid is mutagenic in the Ames Salmonella mutagen test system (Silverman and Andrews, 1977) and causes transformation of Chinese hamster embryo cells in tissue culture (Kesley and Pienta, 1979). Incubation for 30 min with 2.5×10^{-4} M of lithocholic acid can induce single strand breaks in the DNA of mouse lymphoblastoma L1210 cells (Kulkarni et al., 1980).

With this background it is interesting to realize that only the conjugated bile acids originally formed in the liver are present in the germ-free rats and in their excreta. This is in wide contrast to the wide variety of metabolic products in the conventional animals. These studies have led to the present concept that the metabolism of bile acids in the intestines, starting with deconjugation of the amide bonds and the subsequent dehydroxylations, is performed by a series of microorganisms, which must act necessarily in a specific order. It is possible, for example, to demonstrate that no 7α-dehydroxylation of bile acids is carried out by specific microorganism mono-associated in a gnotobiotic animal, if the bile acids are not first deconjugated by other organisms. This reaction cannot be performed by the 7α-dehydroxylating bacteria (Gustafsson et al., 1966). In total, of the 38 bile acid metabolites formed, 34 are the result of microbial activity as shown in Fig. 3.

OTHER XENOBIOTICS AND CARCINOGENS

From recent studies it has become apparent that the intestinal microflora can greatly complicate the metabolism of xenobiotics (Bakke et al., 1980; 1981a and b; Rafter and Nilsson, 1981; Rafter, 1982). When the metabolism of the xenobiotic propachlor was investigated in germ-free rats, a situation similar to that with the bile acid metabolism was demonstrated. Only four metabolites were seen in the faeces, and none of the six methylsulphonylmetabolites excreted by the conventional rats were found in excretions from the germ-free rats (Fig. 4). Faeces from germ-free rats contained only water soluble metabolites (30% of the administered propachlor), whereas faeces from the conventional controls contained nonextractable metabolites (19% of the dose given). Similar influences of the intestinal microflora have been demonstrated in the metabolism of 2-acetamido-4-(chloromethyl)thiazole[3] and pentachloromethylthiobenzene.

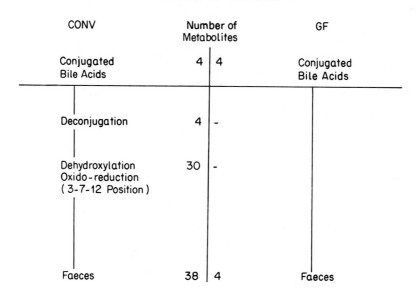

FIG. 3 *Differences in metabolism of bile acids between con-*
ventional (CONV) and germ-free (GF) rats are significant. The
primary bile acids are excreted completely unchanged in the
germ-free rat, whereas a number of metabolites are added by
the action of the intestinal flora in the conventional animal.

   The findings of the studies on the metabolism of xenobiotics in germ-free animals might be summarized as follows:
the xenobiotics chosen in these investigations were selected
because they are known to undergo entero-hepatic circulation,
to be metabolized to mercapturic acid derivatives and to be
excreted in urine and faeces as methylthiols or methyl-
sulphones. In all three cases investigated, such metabolites
were not excreted by the germ-free rats. The intestinal flora
is, thus, responsible for the production of the methyl-
sulphones. Another finding was that the deconjugation of
mercapturates resulted in the production of new metabolites of
xenobiotics. Our studies have also demonstrated that the
intestinal flora is involved in the production of metabolites,
which cannot be extracted from the faeces. Conversely, the
faeces from germ-free rats contained only metabolites which
could be extracted.

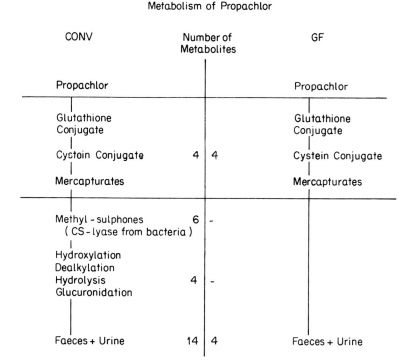

Metabolism of Propachlor

CONV	Number of Metabolites	GF
Propachlor		Propachlor
Glutathione Conjugate		Glutathione Conjugate
Cystoin Conjugate 4	4	Cystein Conjugate
Mercapturates		Mercapturates
Methyl-sulphones 6 (CS-lyase from bacteria)	-	
Hydroxylation Dealkylation Hydrolysis 4 Glucuronidation	-	
Faeces + Urine 14	4	Faeces + Urine

FIG. 4 *When propachlor is introduced in the conventional animal (CONV), the microflora adds 10 metabolites to the 4 produced in the germ-free (GF) rat.*

The important question that now arises is whether these results are applicable to polyaromatic hydrocarbons. Such studies are under way in the author's laboratory concerning the metabolism of benzo(a)pyrene in germ-free and conventional rats.

The physiological importance of the intestinal microflora in the human carcinogenic process is an area which still requires much basic research before any definite relationships are established. The large metabolic capacity of the flora in xenobiotic metabolism, together with the wealth of results obtained from experimental animals, makes it extremely unlikely that the flora has no role to play.

Furthermore, the metabolic events mediating the cancer protecting effects of fibre in the diet, are not known, even

though it has been speculated that these factors beneficially
alter the metabolic activity and/or the composition of the
flora. Thus, by focusing on how these protective factors
alter the metabolic activity, rather than the composition of
the flora by carrying out metabolic studies in germ-free and
conventional animals and by monitoring mutagenicity of germ-
free and conventional excreta, it is hoped that more light can
be thrown on these procedures.

BILE ACIDS, DIETARY FIBRES AND CANCERS

During the past few years there has been intensive discussion
on whether fibres in the diet affect the incidence of colon
cancer in man. In an investigation (Gustafsson and Norman,
1969) to study the influence of fibre content of the diet on
the turnover of bile acids, germ-free and conventional rats
were given three diets: 1) a semisynthetic diet low in fibre,
2) the same diet with 20% pure cellulose added and 3) a commercial diet with a comparatively high fibre content. When
the study was performed in the early 1960s, this content
measured only as the crude fibres was recorded as 4.7%. Recent analyses of this diet by Asp (1982), considering the
present definition of diet fibre as the total non-starch poly-
saccharides and lignin, have given a value of 20.5%, i.e.
close to the amount of pure cellulose added to the semisynthetic diet in this study.

On the first day of the experiment referred to here, 0.1 mg
sodium [24^{14} C] cholate (5 µC) autoclaved in 1 ml water was
given orally to each rat by means of a stomach tube. Through
the same stomach tube, each rat was given a suspension of
100 mg carmine in 1 ml of water.

The elimination rates of cholic acid were always slower in
germ-free than in conventional rats. The addition, however,
of 20% cellulose to the semisynthetic diet D7 shortened the
half-life time of cholic acid, and in animals receiving pellets
it was even shorter than in those on the semisynthetic diets.

The daily excretion of cholic acid and its metabolites was
calculated by dividing the total amount of these compounds
present in the rat by the turnover time. The addition of pure
cellulose to D7 did not increase the bile acid excretion in
either germ-free or conventional rats. Feeding with the
pelleted ration resulted in a significantly higher bile acid
excretion in both the germ-free and conventional animals than
with either of the other two diets tested. In animals receiving the fibre-free diet D7, the germ-free rats had a signfi-
cantly slower bile acid excretion than the conventional rats.
That this is bound to a reduced passage time in the intestinal
tract of germ-free rats was demonstrated by the finding that

carmine was excreted more slowly by germ-free rats than by conventional rats in the groups receiving diet D7 and D7 with cellulose. In germ-free and conventional rats receiving pellets, the same relatively fast excretion of carmine was observed.

Dialysis of faecal homogenates of conventional rats showed that part of the labelled metabolites of cholic acid were excreted in a non-dialysable form. There was a higher excretion of non-dialysable bile acids in rats on pellets than in those on diet D7 + 20% cellulose or D7 alone. There was a much greater proportion of bile acids in the sediment left after centrifugation of the caecal contents in both the germ-free and conventional rats receiving pellets than in those receiving the semisynthetic diet D7.

The different effect of pure cullulose and the fibres in the stock diet in these studies agrees well with the findings of Balmer and Zilversmit (Balmer and Zilversmit, 1974). The conclusions of our studies on the effect of cellulose on bile acid secretion might be summarized as follows:

The amount of bile acids excreted was two to three times higher in both conventional and germ-free rats receiving pellets than in those receiving diet D7. This difference in bile acid secretion between animals receiving different diets cannot, therefore, be caused by an influence of the diet on the gastrointestinal microflora. This effect of the commercial diet could not be due to a high fibre content only, since an increase in the fibre content of the semisynthetic diet D7 by the addition of 20% cellulose did not reproduce the effect obtained with the commercial diet with the same total fibre content. Thus, the properties of the fibres and not the amounts are decisive.

The difference observed in bile acid excretion between germ-free and conventional rats on diet D7 was ascribed mainly to the much longer transit time of intestinal contents in germ-free as compared with conventional rats.

Weisburger *et al.* (1980) have interpreted the effect of dietary fibre in lowering the risk for the development of colon cancer as that of reducing the effect of promoters. Our data merits the conclusion that certain fibres accelerate the intestinal transport of bile acids, not only by their bulk but also through other effects on the colonizing and metabolizing effects of the microflora.

The structure of the fibres for the richness of the flora and the abundant possibilities for an increase in the surface that these fibres provide might be of decisive effect for the action of carcinogens. Recent findings and developments regarding composition, structure and function of the bacterial intestinal flora juxtapositioned to the epithelium and

adjacent structures constitute strong incentives for further
studies.

CONCLUSIONS

When finally judging our personal concept of the relations of
the intestinal microflora to carcinogenesis, the following
problems stand out as worthy of consideration and further work.

1. In the same individual or species the intestinal microflora
in close relationship to the host tissues might be more well
defined and stable than earlier anticipated.
2. The intimate relation of the microbial microflora to the
epithelia in the intestinal tract infers that many results
obtained in microorganisms might be more directly applied to
the cells and tissues.
3. Some carcinogens are not acting as such until metabolized
by the microflora.
4. If such metabolism at one or several steps requires floral
enzymes, the composition of the intestinal microflora might
be of importance when comparing results in animal studies from
different laboratories. Results *in vitro* test systems might
also be influenced by the presence of active microorganisms.

REFERENCES

Aries, V.C., Crowther, J.S., Drasar, B.S., Hill, M.J. and
    Williams, R.E.O. (1969). *Gut* 10, 334-335.
Asp, N.-G. (1982). Personal communication.
Bakke, J.E., Gustafsson, J.-Å. and Gustafsson, B.E. (1980).
    Science 210, 433-435.
Bakke, J.E., Aschbacher, P.W., Feil, V.J. and Gustafsson, B.E.
    (1981a). *Xenobiotica* 11, 173-178.
Bakke, J.E., Rafter, J.J., Lindeskog, P., Feil, V.J.,
    Gustafsson, J.-Å. and Gustafsson, B.E. (1981b). *Biochem.
    Pharmacol.* 30, 1839-1844.
Balmer, J. and Zilversmit, D.B. (1974). *J. Nutr.* 104, 1319-
    1328.
Finegold, S.M. (1970). *Delaware Med. J.* 42, 341-345, 350.
Gustafsson, B.E. (1948). *Acta Pathol. Microbiol. Scand.*
    Suppl. 73, 1-130. Doctoral Thesis.
Gustafsson, B.E. and Norman, A. (1969). *Br. J. Nutr.* 23,
    429-442.
Gustafsson, B.E. and Norin, K.E. (1977). *Acta Pathol. Micro-
    biol. Scand.* 85, 1-8.
Gustafsson, B.E., Midtvedt, T. and Norman, A. (1966). *J. Exp.
    Med.* 123, 413-432.
Gustafsson, B.E. and Maunsbach, A.B. (1971). *Z. Zellforsch*
    120, 555-578.

Gustafsson, B., Gustafsson, J.-Å. and Carlstedt-Duke, B.
    (1977). *Acta Med. Scand.* 201, 155-160.
Kesley, M.I. and Pienta, R.J. (1979). *Cancer Lett.* 6, 143-
    149.
Kulkarni, M.S., Heiderpriem, P.M. and Yiedling, K. (1980).
    Cancer Res. 40, 2666-2669.
Laqueur, G.L. (1964). *Fed. Proc.* 23, 1386-1387.
Laqueur, G.L., McDaniel, E.G. and Matsumoto, H. (1967). *J.
    Nat. Cancer Inst.* 39, 355-371.
Luckey, T.D. (1977). *Am. J. Clin. Nutr.* 30, 1753-1761.
Midtvedt, T. and Gustafsson, B.E. (1981). *Current Microbiol.*
    6, 13-15.
Narisawa, T., Magadia, N.E., Weisburger, J.H. and Wynder, E.L.
    (1974). *J. Nat. Cancer Inst.* 55, 1093-1097.
Pollard, M. and Luckert, P.H. (1979). *Lab. Animal Sci.* 29,
    74-77.
Rafter, J.J. and Nilsson, L. (1981). *Xenobiotica* 11, 771-778.
Rafter, J.J. (1982). Doctoral Thesis.
Reddy, B.S., Narisawa, T., Weisburger, J.H. and Wynder, E.L.
    (1976). *J. Nat. Cancer Inst.* 56, 441-442.
Reddy, B.S., Watanabe, K., Weisburger, J.H. and Wynder, E.L.
    (1977). *Cancer Res.* 37, 3238-3242.
Reyniers, J.A., Trexler, P.C., Ervin, R.F., Wagner, M.,
    Luckey, T.D. and Gordon, H.A. (1949). *In* Lobund Report
    No.2, pp.1-116. Univ. of Notre Dame Press, Paris.
Silverman, S.J. and Andrews, A.W. (1977). *J. Nat. Cancer
    Inst.* 59, 1557-1559.
Spatz, M., McDaniel, E.G. and Laqueur, G.L. (1966). *Proc.
    Soc. Exp. Biol. and Med.* 121, 417-422.
Weisburger, J.H., Reddy, B.S., Hill, P., Cohen, L.A., Wynder,
    E.L. and Spingarn, N.E. (1980). *Bull. N.Y. Acad. Sci.*
    56, 673-696.

CHANGING TRENDS IN CARCINOGENESIS

I. Berenblum

The Weizmann Institute of Science, Rehovot, Israel

Scientific progress can be measured in different ways; there
is, for instance, the encyclopaedic approach, facilitated
nowadays by computerized storage of information. Its weakness
lies in trivial contributions outweighing and obscuring the
more important ones, thus tending to impede rather than expe-
dite the evaluation of scientific events. In any case, the
mere compilation and classification of data, "letting the facts
speak for themselves", is not the best way to explain basic
principles.

There is, alternatively, the inclination to stress dramatic
discoveries which manage, in one go, to solve certain out-
standing problems and, at the same time, open up new avenues
of research. This approach suffers from the opposite tendency
of neglecting the gradual accumulation of significant information that can sometimes have as important an impact on
scientific progress as the more spectacular kind of breakthrough. Even a highly successful breakthrough is, after all,
but a stepping-stone in a progressive trend, based on earlier
information and leading to future discoveries.

The task of the analyst, trying to interpret the significance of scientific discoveries, is itself precarious. Histor-
ians, trained in objective analysis of the past, tend to focus
attention on early discoveries, from times of ancient Greece
to the nineteenth century, rather than on recent progress in
science. Practising scientists, on the other hand, are too
much taken up with exciting contemporary advances to be able
to judge dispassionately the real importance of the latest
discoveries in historical perspective. There is, thus, the
strong temptation among us to base our judgement on the latest
findings and to consider earlier contributions unimportant,

THEORIES AND MODELS
IN CELLULAR TRANSFORMATION

without at least attempting to explain why the latter are no
longer valid or relevant.

In trying to evaluate the progress in the field of carcinogenesis, I hope to avoid this pitfall by paying particular
attention to changing trends over the years, and looking for
the reasons why so many popular lines of enquiry have passed
into eclipse or have even become completely forgotten by contemporary investigators.

Pathologists and clinicians have always recognized the clear
distinction and, at the same time, the important interrelation-
ship, between aetiology, i.e. the causes of disease, and pathogenesis, i.e. the way tissues respond to their action. It is,
therefore, surprising that in the case of carcinogenesis the
two have, until recent times, been kept isolated from one
another.

Consider, for instance, the various theories about cancer
development put forward during the pre-experimental and early
experimental times. Those that dealt with causative factors,
e.g. the "irritation theory", failed to explain why non-
specific damage to tissues should lead to the development of
cancer, the assumption being that cancerous growth was a mere
exaggeration of reparative hyperplasia in response to injury.
On the other hand, the theories that dealt with the problem
from the viewpoint of tissue response, e.g. the "embryonal
rest" theory, or that of "disturbed tissue equilibrium", or
later, Warburg's theory of "disturbed carbohydrate metabolism",
paid little attention to causative factors that might have
been responsible for the postulated disturbances. (For a
critical analysis of these outmoded theories, see Berenblum
(1974).)

The situation naturally improved with the introduction of
animal experiments for the study of carcinogenesis. Instead
of building speculative theories, mainly based on faulty
analogies with non-neoplastic processes, as was the case previously, reliance could now be placed on results of controlled
experiments. The course of progress was, nevertheless, beset
with obstacles of a technical nature, which made it very often
difficult to carry out the really crucial experiments, and
many of the interim conclusions had subsequently to be aban-
doned.

Such a predicament arose at the very start, with the use
of coal tar for experimental tumour induction. During the
heyday of tar carcinogenesis, from 1915 to 1930, more than
600 research publications on the subject appeared in the
literature (see reviews by Woglom, 1926; Watson, 1932; Seelig
and Cooper, 1933). Contemporary investigators are hardly
familiar with any part of this early intensive effort. Apart
from the usual lack of interest in earlier work there are at

least two valid reasons for the failure of tar carcinogenesis to have had any important impact on subsequent work: (1) carcinogenicity studies with tar were virtually restricted to skin applications, toxicity considerations rendering the material unsuitable for *systemic* carcinogenesis. *In vitro* was not even thought of then; and (2) coal tar, being a complex mixture of hundreds of components, made it impossible for investigators to differentiate between the biological side-effects that might have had a bearing on the carcinogenic process, and those side-effects that were unrelated to the dominant action and, therefore, irrelevant to the problem concerned with the mechanism of carcinogenic action.

To overcome these limitations a group of investigators in London, under the guidance of E.L. Kennaway, succeeded in isolating in crystalline form an active principle of tar: the polycyclic aromatic hydrocarbon, benzpyrene (Cook *et al.*, 1933), thus placing experimental carcinogenicity on a sound scientific footing.

The immediate result of this important achievement was to embark on an extensive programme of chemical synthesis of compounds related to benzpyrene hoping that the relationship between the chemical structure of carcinogens and their potencies of action would provide a clue to the mechanism of tumour induction.

Though the information thus acquired (see reviews by Cook and Kennaway, 1938; 1940) was of inestimable value to subsequent research in experimental carcinogenesis, the underlying idea of trying to explain the *biological* process of carcinogenesis in terms of *chemical* properties of the inciting agents, was not only over-ambitious but also fundamentally faulty. While this programme of chemical synthesis was still under way information began to accumulate that rendered the idea of a close link between chemical structure and carcinogenic potency virtually untenable.

First was the discovery of other kinds of carcinogens totally unrelated to the polycyclic aromatic hydrocarbons, e.g. of oestrone, carcinogenic for mammary tissue; aminoazo-compounds, carcinogenic for the liver; somewhat later, carbon tetrachloride, carcinogenic for the liver; urethane, carcinogenic for the lungs, etc. It did not require much knowledge of chemical structure to appreciate the extraordinary diversity of compounds capable of producing tumours (see Fig. 1). This is apart from ionizing radiation also being carcinogenic.

As for attempts to quantitate carcinogenic potency, this also ran into difficulties. Apart from the inability of comparing effects of skin application with those resulting from subcutaneous injection or systemic administration, the results also varied enormously according to the species of animals

Carcinogen	Formula	Class of Compound	Organ Response
3:4-Benzpyrene or Benzo(a)pyrene	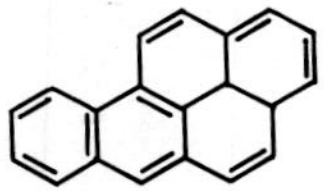	Polycyclic aromatic hydrocarbons	Most organs and tissues in the body
"Butter yellow" (4-Dimethylamino-azobenzene)	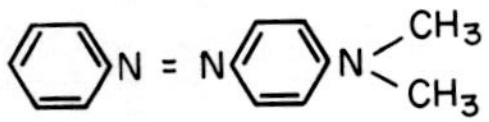 $N = N - N \diagdown \begin{smallmatrix} CH_3 \\ CH_3 \end{smallmatrix}$	Synthetic dye "intermediates"	Liver
Beta-naphthylamine	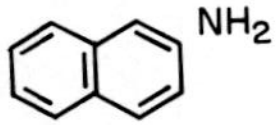 NH_2	Synthetic dye "intermediate"	Urinary bladder
Urethane (ethyl-carbamate)	$NH_2 - \overset{O}{\underset{\parallel}{C}} - O - C_2H_5$	Carbamates	Lungs: less commonly other organs
Carbon tetrachloride	CCl_4	Chlorinated aliphatic hydrocarbons	Liver

FIG. 1

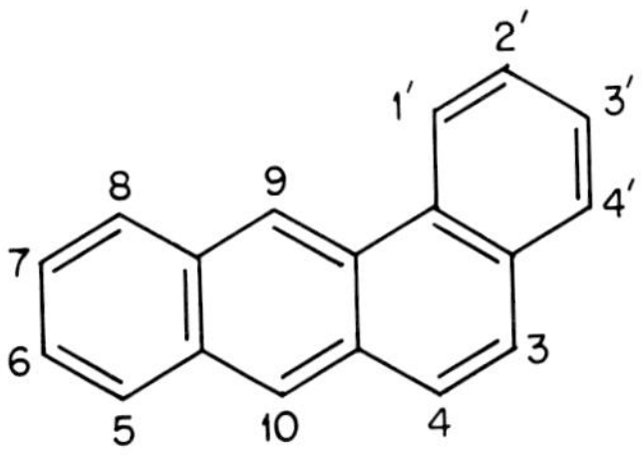

(Old numbering)

1'-Me = -	5-Me = +
2'-Me = -	6-Me = ++
3'-Me = -	7-Me = +
4'-Me = -	8-Me = -
3-Me = -	9-Me = +++
4-Me = +	10-Me = ++++

FIG. 2 *Carcinogenicity of methyl derivatives of 1:2-benzanthracene.*

used for testing or the tissues acted upon. The most potent carcinogens, under one set of conditions, might prove to be non-carcinogenic under different conditions. Some investigators were naturally troubled from the start by the anomalous situation where, whereas no similarity in structure could be discerned among the various classes of carcinogens, there was nevertheless a striking degree of chemical specificity within each class of compounds. This was particularly evident among the methyl derivatives of benzanthracene, where a change in position of the methyl group could convert an effective carcinogen into a totally inactive one (see Fig. 2).

With hindsight, we are now able to account for the apparent conflict between chemical diversity versus specificity of carcinogenic action, and the fact that chemically *non-reactive* compounds like the polycyclic aromatic hydrocarbons could function at all as carcinogens. The explanation, as we know it now, is that most of the carcinogens are in fact "pro-carcinogens", which have to be enzymically activated, i.e. metabolized, in the body into "ultimate carcinogens" before being able to react with essential elements within the living cell, as a primary step in carcinogenesis (see review by Miller and Miller, 1981; Conney, 1982).

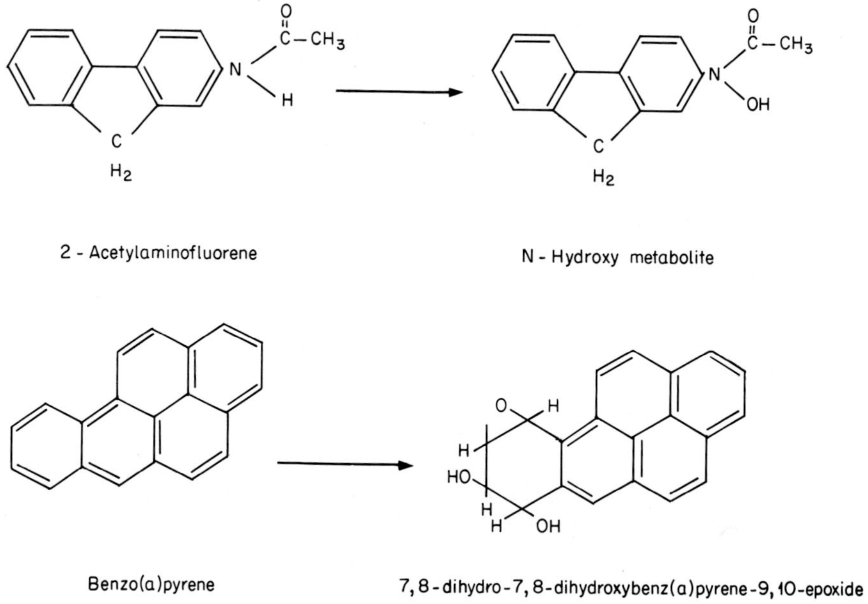

2 - Acetylaminofluorene

N - Hydroxy metabolite

Benzo(a)pyrene

7,8-dihydro-7,8-dihydroxybenz(a)pyrene-9,10-epoxide

FIG. 3 *Metabolic activation of procarcinogens.*

Attempts were, in fact, made early on to determine the
metabolic fate of polycyclic aromatic hydrocarbons in the body
(see Biochemical Society Symposium, 1950). The early results
were, from the viewpoint of carcinogenesis, disappointing and
frustrating, in that the identified metabolites were all detoxication products, and thus not involved in the carcinogenic process. Further work along these lines was, for a long
time, in abeyance, until important advances in analytical
methods made it possible to re-examine the problem, resulting
in the detection and identification of active metabolites,
e.g. of *N*-hydroxy derivatives of amino aromatic compounds
(Cramer *et al.*, 1960), and of the bay-region dihydrodiol epox-
ides of polycyclic aromatic hydrocarbons (Sims *et al.*, 1974)
(see Fig. 3). Such metabolic studies are now being vigorously
pursued, with the newer methodology extended to other classes
of carcinogens.

Anticipating the actual identification of the "ultimate"
carcinogens, much information already existed about the
ability of carcinogenic hydrocarbons (or rather their unidentified metabolic products) to bind with DNA, RNA, and
proteins *in vivo* (Miller and Miller, 1952; Heidelberger and

Moldenhauer, 1956; etc.). Realization of the crucial significance of DNA binding came later, with the accumulated evidence
of a mutational change in the cell as an essential feature of
neoplastic transformation (Knudsen, 1973; Trosko and Chu, 1975;
Hewitt *et al.*, 1979). The logical inference of all this was
that simple alkylating agents should be able to act as carcinogens without necessarily undergoing prior metabolic activation,
and this was, in fact, found to be the case (Brookes and Lawley,
1964; Brookes, 1975).

The theory of a cell mutation as the cause of cancer,
initially based on plausible but purely speculative reasoning,
is quite an ancient one (cf. Bauer, 1928). Its revival, in a
retriced form, came partly as an outcome of the metabolic
studies already referred to, but also from earlier experiments
of a biological kind, which arose from two contemporaneous
series of experiments pointing to independent stages, or components, of carcinogenesis (Rous and Kidd, 1941; Berenblum,
1941) now generally known as "the two-stage, initiation-
promotion, mechanism of carcinogenesis". What is particularly
relevant to the present discussion is the reason for the long
delay - more than two decades - from the initial formulation
of the initiation-promotion theory to its present acceptance
as a dominant feature of carcinogenic action.

Let us consider for a moment what information was already
available about the subject from the start, what technical
obstacles had to be overcome to proceed in order to determine
the actual mechanisms of the component phases, and what other
considerations played a part in "popularizing" the initiation-
promotion principle.

The information available at the start, i.e. in the 1940s,
was already quite extensive, including the fact that initiating
action was a rapid process, causing an irreversible change in
the cell. The implication that this might involve a change
in the chromosomal make-up of the cell was not seriously taken
up by us at the time. Only much later, with the biochemical
evidence of DNA binding, did it become apparent that the
initiating component of the two-stage process was, indeed,
dependent on a mutational change, in contrast to the slow
promoting component, which clearly consisted of some kind of
epigenetic action.

Thus, while the mechanism of tumour initiation eventually
began to be understood, the mechanism of tumour promotion
continued to be a mystery. Why, in fact, was promoting action
needed at all?

The fact that a gene mutation, producing a *dormant* tumour
cell, needed some kind of "awakening" process for effective
neoplastic expression, was in itself not so surprising. After
all, if a *normal* gene can remain inactive, requiring a

complicated "switching-on" process (cf. Jacob and Monod, 1961), so surely might a *tumour-type* mutation. What could not be taken for granted, however, was that the epigenetic tumour promotion process involved a similar kind of action.

One of the main reasons for the slow progress (and, for that matter, the general lack of interest for so long a period) in two-stage carcinogenesis, was the fact that the only effective promoting agent at the time, croton oil, was a complex mixture of indeterminate nature, and active only on mouse skin. (We see here a close parallel to the situation earlier on, with respect to tar carcinogenesis. There was, indeed, little chance of progress being made until chemically pure promoters became available.)

The successful isolation and identification of the active principle of croton oil as 12-O-tetradecanoylphorbol-13-acetate, or TPA (also known as phorbol myristate acetate, or PMA), by two independent groups (see Hecker, 1968; Van Duren, 1969), and the availability of related compounds possessing varying potencies of tumour promoting activity (Fig. 4) heralded a great intensification of effort throughout the world in the experimental study of the mechanism of tumour promotion. At the same time, the discovery of other kinds of tumour promoters, many of them acting systemically and affecting different organs and tissues other than the skin, greatly extended the scope of research in the field.

As a measure of the new interest in the mechanism of tumour promotion, close to 2,000 publications on the subject appeared during the past three years alone, as listed in the monthly abstracts of ICRDB Cancerogram series on Modifications of Carcinogenesis (1979-1983). The fact that we are still a long way from understanding how tumour promotion operates, calls for some explanation.

The currently most common approach to the problem is based on correlative studies between potencies of tumour promotion, among a series of phorbol esters, and other properties they happen to possess, in the hope that a good fit might throw light on the mechanism of promoting action (Boutwell, 1974; Weinstein *et al.*, 1979; see also the various contributions in Hecker *et al.*, 1980). Two points of criticism may be levelled against too much reliance being put on the outcome of this kind of approach: (1) the over-abundance of seemingly good fits observed (see Table 1), and (2) the high probability of chance associations, as against meaningful interdependence, when dealing with such small numbers of compounds for comparison.

There is, in any case, a strong likelihood of two different and independent forms of tumour promotion: (1) that involved in the change-over from the quiescent to the proliferative

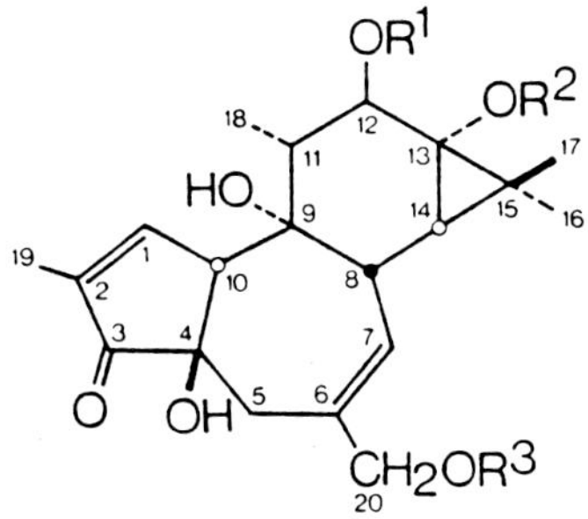

Compounds	Promoting Activity on Mouse Skin
Phorbol (unesterified 1.e. $R_1=R_2=R_3=H$)	$\pm$
12,13-Diesters of phorbol ($R_1=R_2=$acyl, $R_3=H$)	
12-0-Tetradecanoylphorbol-13-acetate (TPA)	++++
Phorbol-12,13-didecanoate	+++
Phorbol-12,13-dobenzoate	+++
Phorbol-12,13-dibutyrate	++
Phorbol-12,13-diacetate	+
4-0-Methyl-TPA	$\pm$
Phorbol-12-tetradecanoate (TP)	–
Phorbol-13-tetradecanoate (PT)	++
4α-phorbol-12,13-didecanoate	–
12,13,20-triesters of phorbol ($R_1=R_2=R_3=$acyl)	
Various triesters	–

(Hecker, personal communication)

FIG. 4 *Tumour promoting properties of phorbol derivatives.*

state (as in the development of a benign tumour), possibly functioning at the "operon" level in the nucleus; and (2) the endowment of invasive and other malignant properties, possibly associated with changes in the cell surface membrane (Berenblum and Armuth, 1981).

Apart from the intensification of effort in laboratory

TABLE 1

*Correlations of Potencies of Promoting Action
with Other Properties (Side-effects) of Phorbol Esters*

A. IN MOUSE SKIN

1. Hyperplasia and inflammatory reactions.

2. Increased DNA, RNA and protein synthesis.

3. Changes in electrophoretic profile of a protein fraction.

4. Increased synthesis of phospholipids, histones, prosta-
glandins, etc.

5. Increased ornithine decarboxylase (ODC) activity.

6. Increased protease activity.

7. Changes in cyclic AMP and GMP activities.

8. Induction of "dark cells".

B. EFFECTS ON CELLS IN TISSUE CULTURE

1. Decreased mobility of cells.

2. Loss of gap junctions of epidermal cells.

3. Decreased amounts of LETS proteins in chick embryo
fibroblasts.

C. SOME OTHER EFFECTS

1. Changes in metabolic behaviour of leucocytes and lymphocytes.

2. Stimulation of platelet aggregation.

3. Changes in sea urchin development.

---

research, renewed interest in the problem of initiation-
promotion also arose from clinical evidence of multiple factors in human carcinogenesis (Higginson, 1980; Peto, 1982).
But as so often happens during peak periods of popularity,
this gave rise to certain claims that seemed unwarranted,
particularly with multiple factors operating systemically,
where one could not easily distinguish between true initiation-
promotion and other forms of cocarcinogenesis.

TABLE 2
Highest and Lowest Incidences of Cancer in Different Organs

Organ	Highest	Lowest	Differential*
Oesophagus	Northern Iran	Israel	x 300
Skin	Australia	India	> 200
Liver	Mosambique	Norway	x 100
Bronchus and lung	England	Central Africa	x 50
Nasal passages	Singapore (Chinese)	England	x 40
Prostate	USA (blacks)	Japan	x 40
Mouth	India	Denmark	x 25
Stomach	Japan	Uganda	x 25
Colon and Rectum	Denmark	Central Africa	x 25
Pancreas	Switzerland	India	x 15
Uterus	Colombia	Israel	x 15
Breast	USA and Europe	Japan	x 8
Thyroid	Switzerland	England	x 5
Leukaemia	USA	India	x 5

* These are approximate estimates, but give an idea of the wide range of variations for some of the more important types of cancer in man.

The existence of other forms of cocarcinogenesis has been known for a long time (Berenblum, 1969); but with so much concern nowadays with initiation-promotion, these other influences tend to be bypassed or overlooked. The distinction is nevertheless important, both on theoretical grounds and as a guide to cancer prevention in man.

From epidemiological studies the incidences of specific forms of cancer differ very much according to geographical location (see Table 2). From this, and other findings, it appears that some 80-90% of all human cancers are in some way environmental in origin. Since many of these influences are known not to be carcinogenic when acting alone, it is tempting to suppose that they function as promoting agents, superimposed on unidentified initiators. Yet this is not always the case.

TABLE 3

Co-carcinogenic Influences other than Tumour Production

---

1. Facilitating nitrosation of secondary amines *in vivo*.
2. Affecting the balance between activation and detoxication of procarcinogens.
3. Affecting enzymic repaid of damaged DNA.
4. Changing the sensitivity of cells to carcinogenic action.
5. Involvement of hormonal or immunological homeostatic mechanisms.
6. Possible determinants of viral oncogenesis.

Consider, for instance, (1) the interaction of nitrites with secondary amines *in vivo*, resulting in the production of carcinogenic nitrosamines, the process capable of being inhibited by vitamins C and E; (2) factors influencing the balance between activation and detoxication of procarcinogens; (3) conditions affecting enzymic repair of damaged DNA; (4) changes in sensitivity of cells to carcinogenic action; (5) homeostatic mechanisms of tumour development; and (6) possible determinants of viral oncogenesis (Table 3). All these might profoundly affect the outcome of potential carcinogenic action, without functioning as promoters, in the sense of "awakening" dormant tumour cells.

The homeostatic mechanisms, both hormonal and immunological, call for special consideration. Hormonal control operates most effectively at the post-promoting phase, during early growth in a hormone-dependent tumour (Foulds, 1969). Hormonal influences can, however, also be demonstrated experimentally during the promoting phase of carcinogenesis (Furth, 1982; Armstrong, 1982); and can, in theory, even affect the initiating phase, insofar as mutagenic action is most pronounced in proliferating tissues during mitotic division (Iversen, 1974), which is itself, in many instances, under hormonal influence.

It seems, however, that homeostatic hormonal control is not of major importance in carcinogenesis, and is, in any case, largely restricted to tumour induction in tissues that are normally under strong hormonal influence.

The homeostatic immunological control of carcinogenesis — known as the "immunosurveillance theory of tumour development" (Thomas, 1959; Burnet, 1964; Good and Finstad, 1969) once held in high esteem, has, in the light of subsequent analysis (Prehn, 1971; Baldwin, 1973; Allison, 1975) been found to have serious limitations.

Based on the discovery of tumour-specific antigens, appearing even in connection with autochthonous, carcinogen-induced, primary tumours (Foley, 1953), the immunosurveillance theory postulated that the body was capable of immunologically destroying tumour cells during their early stages of appearance (i.e. essentially as dormant tumour cells), and that only those cells that somehow escaped the "immunological barrier" developed into progressively growing tumours. While the theory is still a debatable issue, it now seems that immunosurveillance might, under certain conditions, effectively operate in connection with virus-induced tumours (Möller and Möller, 1975), but probably plays an insignificant role in other forms of tumour induction and development.

One of the most striking examples of "changing trends in carcinogenesis" is related to the role of viruses in tumour induction. The "virus theory of cancer", it will be remembered, was initially a hypothetical concept, to account for the failure to detect microorganisms in human tumours, at a time when bacteria were found to be responsible for so many other diseases. Then came two critical discoveries by Ellerman and Bang (1908) and by Rous (1911) of the transmission, by filtrates free from cells or bacteria, of a fowl leukaemia and a fowl sarcoma, respectively.

This might well have stimulated world-wide interest in what appeared to be a major breakthrough in the search for the cause(s) of cancer, but for the introduction, soon after, of chemical (tar) carcinogenesis that seemed, at the time, to conflict radically with viral carcinogenesis. What actually happened was the creation of two independent schools of thought: a minority favouring the viral origin of cancer and a majority firmly attached to a chemical causative mechanism, each group virtually ignoring the work of the other.

Two leading exponents of the viral theory, during the 1940s, were Oberling (1944) and Duran-Reynals (1952), who valiantly fought for the important role of viruses in tumour causation. The sad fact was that appropriate techniques for the study of viral properties, composition and behaviour were not available at the time. These early investigators were, for that reason, fighting a losing battle. Yet further examples of viral transmission were already known at the time e.g. the Shope papilloma virus in rabbits (Shope and Hurst, 1933); the mouse mammary tumour virus (Bittner, 1940); and the mouse leukaemia virus (Gross, 1951).

The re-emergence of research on viral participation in carcinogenesis, facilitated by new advances in technique, developed along three independent lines: (1) *in vivo* studies, with particular emphasis on leukaemogenesis (Kaplan, 1967;

Haran-Ghera, 1980); (2) neoplastic transformation by viruses
in vitro (Dulbecco, 1957); and (3) studies of mechanisms of
viral action at the molecular level (Klein, 1982).

One of the difficulties of reconciling viral and chemical
carcinogenesis was the fact that causative viruses tended to
persist and replicate in the induced tumours, being apparently
responsible for the continued neoplastic behaviour of the
tumours, whereas chemical causative agents soon disappeared
from the body and thus played no part in the behaviour of the
transformed cells.

When chemical carcinogens were shown to function as mutagens by interacting with the DNA of the cell, the idea emerged
that portions of the DNA viruses might be incorporated into
the DNA genome of the cell. According to this scheme, the
distinction between chemical and viral action was narrowed
down, with chemical carcinogens producing a change in the
genetic make-up of the cell while viruses provided added
genetic information.

The scheme, thus far, might be represented as in Fig. 5.
There was still the problem of RNA tumour viruses, but this
was eventually solved by the discovery of reverse transcription of RNA viruses into DNA proviruses (Temin, 1974).

Then came the postulated "oncogene theory" in its original
form of cancer (Huebner and Todaro, 1969), claiming the

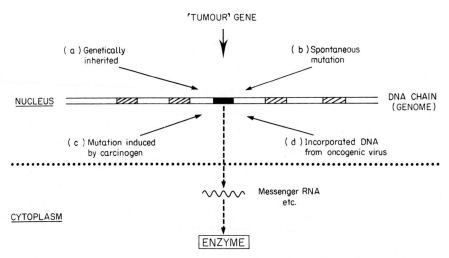

FIG. 5 *Mechanism of tumour induction through a change in
DNA composition.*

existence of such genes as *normal* components of cells, alleg-
edly capable, under certain conditions, of liberating into the
cytoplasm "C-type virus particles" that could act as tumour
viruses. The scheme, based initially on indirect evidence,
has since received support in a modified form by refined
immunological procedures; while more recently, with the use
of recombinant technology, a close chemical relationship has
been established between certain normally-occurring genes and
viral elements; such genes also capable of being activated by
chromosomal translocation (Klein, 1982).

The final reconciliation between physical, chemical and
viral carcinogenesis may still be far ahead, though we seem
to be approaching that goal, and thereby satisfying one's
natural inclination of assuming the existence of a unified
mechanism of carcinogenesis.

Reverting to factors influencing chemical carcinogenesis,
the study of anticarcinogenic action has been receiving increasing attention in recent years (Wattenburg, 1977; 1980;
Van Duuren and Melchionne, 1969) with particular emphasis on
their modes of action. There are two important considerations
in this connection: (1) the need for discovering anticarcinogens that are free from toxic side-effects, and (2) knowledge
about their manner of action during the long latent period of
carcinogenesis (Lotan, 1980; Sporn and Newton, 1981).

The two problems are in a sense interrelated, for the more
one knows about the mechanism of anticarcinogenic action, the
better the prospects of discovering non-toxic agents (as
against unplanned tests by trial and error).

Some anticarcinogens are known to act, by virtue of their
antioxidant properties, by interfering with the enzymic activation of procarcinogens, i.e. at the pre-initiating phase of
carcinogenesis. Not much concrete evidence is available about
anticarcinogens operating actually during the initiating phase,
though one could envisage such interfering mechanisms. The
most hopeful scheme of anticarcinogenic action, from the viewpoint of cancer prevention, is that which might operate during
the long latent period of carcinogenesis i.e. acting as anti-
promoting agents.

In this connection, attention should be drawn to the growing
interest in the effect of diet on carcinogenesis from at least
three directions: (1) inhibition of tumour induction by non-
specific caloric restriction of an otherwise balanced diet;
(2) the important role of fats, especially in connection with
mammary carcinogenesis; and (3) factors affecting the metabolic conversion of bile acids and of cholesterol, into potential promoting agents, notably in connection with carcinogenesis of the colon.

In the case of high fat diets this has been traced to

unsaturated fatty acids, notably linoleic acid; and while generally thought to operate through induced changes in the hormonal balance in the body, e.g. of prolactin and oestrogens, alternative mechanisms have recently been suggested as more likely (Welsch and Aylsworth, 1983). The final solution of the problem will undoubtedly have a profound impact on the possible prevention of breast cancer in humans.

From the viewpoint of multi-stage carcinogenesis contemporary studies are, as already indicated, focused on: (1) the metabolic conversion of "procarcinogens" into "ultimate carcinogens"; (2) the binding of these activated metabolites with DNA receptors in the cell; and (3) the precise mechanism of action of tumour promoters. Far less attention is being paid nowadays to co-carcinogenic effects that play no part in multi-stage carcinogenesis or which influence it in an indirect way only.

I shall resist the temptation of trying to extrapolate the finding of the past in order to predict changing trends in years to come. One could, of course, point to those aspects that have been fairly well explored, and predict a slackening of effort in those fields in the future. One could likewise stress those areas that are still in process of exploration, and predict an intensification of effort in those fields. What cannot be foretold is the unexpected new discoveries that are likely to change radically the present trends.

As for the overall assessment of experimental carcinogenesis during the past seven decades of endeavour, the progress made is undoubtedly impressive, in spite of, or perhaps encouraged by, the changes in trends discussed in this review. Progress in any branch of science can be said to reach maturity when theoretical principles begin to have practical application. In this sense, carcinogenesis would seem to have reached the threshold of maturity.

REFERENCES

Allison, A.C. (1975). "Immunological Surveillance Against Tumour Cells. *In* Cancer: A Comprehensive Treatise" (Ed. F.F. Becker), Vol.4, pp.237-258. Plenum Press, New York.
Armstrong, B. (1982). Endocrine Factors in Human Carcinogenesis. IARC Monogram 39, Host Factors in Human Carcinogenesis. 193-221. International Agency for Research on Cancer, Lyon.
Baldwin, R.W. (1973). *Advanc. Cancer Res.* 18, 1-75.
Bauer, K.H. (1928). "Mutationstheorie der Geschwulst-Entstehung". Julius Springer, Berlin.
Berenblum, I. (1941). *Cancer Res.* 1, 807-814.
Berenblum, I. (1969). *Progr. Exp. Tumor Res.* 11, 21-30.

Berenblum, I. (1974). "Carcinogenesis as a Biological Problem"
North-Holland Publishing Co., Amsterdam.

Berenblum, I. and Armuth, V. (1981). *Biochim. Biophys. Acta*
651, 51-63.
Biochemical Society Symposium No.5 (1950). Biological Oxidation of Aromatic Rings. Cambridge University Press,
England.
Bittner, J.J. (1940). *Am. J. Cancer* 39, 104-113.
Boutwell, R.K. (1974). *CRC Crit. Rev. Toxicol.* 2, 419-444.
Brookes, P. (1975). *Life Sciences* 16, 331-344.
Brookes, P. and Lawley, P.D. (1964). *Br. Med. Bull.* 20, 91-95.
Burnet, R.M. (1964). *Br. Med. Bull.* 20, 154-158.
Conney, A.H. (1982). *Cancer Res.* 42, 4875-4917.
Cook, J.W. and Kennaway, E.L. (1939). *Am. J. Cancer* 33, 50-97.
Cook, J.W. and Kennaway, E.L. (1940). *Am. J. Cancer* 39, 381-582.
Cook, J.W., Hewitt, C.L. and Hieger, I. (1933). *J. Chem. Soc.*
pp. 395-405.
Cramer, J.W., Miller, J.A. and Miller, E.C. (1960). *J. Biol.
Chem.* 235, 885-888.
Dulbecco, R. (1975). *Cold Spring Harbor Smpy. Quant. Biol.*
39, 1-6.
Duran-Reynals, F. (1952). *Ann. N.Y. Acad. Sci.* 54, 977-991.
Ellerman, V. and Bang, O. (1908). *Zbt. Bakt.* 46, 595-609.

Foulds, L. (1969). "Neoplastic Development". Academic Press,
London & New York.
Foley, E.J. (1953). *Cancer Res.* 13, 835-837.
Furth, J. (1982). *In* "Hormones as Etiological Agents in Neoplasia. In "Cancer: A Comprehensive Treatise" (Ed. F.F.
Becker), Vol.1 (2nd edition), pp.89-134. Plenum Press,
New York.
Good, R.A. and Finstad, J. (1969). Essential Relationship
between the Lymphoid System, Immunity and Malignancy.
National Cancer Institute Monogr., 31, 41-85.

Gross, L. (1951). *Proc. Soc. Exp. Biol. Med.* 76, 27-32.
Haran-Ghera, N. (1980). *In* "Viral Oncology" (Ed. G. Klein),
pp.161-185.
Hecker, E. (1968). *Cancer Res.* 28, 2338-2349.
Hecker, E., Fusenig, N.E., Kunz, W., Marks, F. and Thielmann,
H.W. (Eds.) (1982). "Carcinogenesis. A Comprehensive Survey"
Vol.7.
Heidelberger, C. and Moldenhauer, M.G. (1956). *Cancer Res.*
16, 442-449.
Hewitt, R.R., Harless, J., Lloyd, R.S., Love, J. and

Robberson, D.L. (1979). *In* "Carcinogens: Identification and Molecular Action" (Eds. A.C. Griffin and C.R. Shaw), pp.107-120. Raven Press, New York.

Higginson, J. (1980). *J. Environm. Pathol. Toxicol.* 3, 113-125.

Huebner, R.J. and Todaro, G.J. (1969). *Proc. Natl. Acad. Sci. USA* 64, 1087-1094.

ICRDB Cancergram, Series CK04: Modification of Carcinogens (1979-1983), US Department of Health, Education and Welfare.

Iversen, O.H. (1974). Cell proliferation kinetics and Carcinogenesis: A Review. Proc. 5th Internat. Symp. on Biological Characterization of Human Tumours. (Eds. D. Davis and C. Maltoni) pp.21-29. Excerpta Medica, Amsterdam.

Jacob, F. and Monod, J. (1961). *Cold Spring Harbor Symp. Quant. Biol.* 26, 193-211.

Kaplan, H.S. 1967. *Cancer Res.* 27, 1325-1340.

Klein, G. (1982). "Advances in Viral Oncology" Vol.1, Raven Press, New York.

Knudsen, A.G. Jr. (1973). *Advanc. Cancer Res.* 17, 317-352.

Lotan, R. (1980). *Biochim. Biophys. Acta* 605, 33-91.

Miller, E.C. and Miller, J.A. (1952). *Cancer Res.* 12, 547-556.

Miller, E.C. and Miller, J.A. (1981). *Cancer* 47, 1055-1064.

Möller, G. and Möller, E. (1975). *J. Natl. Cancer Inst.* 55, 755-759.

Oberling, C. (1944). The Riddle of Cancer. (Trans. by W.H. Woglom), Yale Univ. Press, New Haven.

Peto, R. (1982). Carcinogenesis as a Multistage Process - Evidence for Human Studies. IARC Monogr. 39: Factors in Human Carcinogenesis. pp.27-28. Internat. Agency for Research on Cancer. Lyon.

Prehn, R.T. (1971). *Progr. Exp. Tumor Res.* 14, 1-24.

Rous, P. (1911). *J. Exp. Med.* 13, 397-411.

Rous, P. and Kidd, J.G. (1941). *J. Exp. Med.* 73, 365-390.

Seelig, M.G. and Cooper, Z.K. (1933). *Am. J. Cancer* 17, 589-667.

Shope, R.E. and Hurst, E.W. (1933). *J. Exp. Med.* 38, 607-624.

Sims, P., Grover, P.L., Swaisland, A., Pal, K. and Hewer, A. (1974). *Nature* 252, 326-328.

Sporn, M.B. and Newton, D.L. (1981). *In* "Inhibition of Tumor Induction and Development" (Eds. S. Zadeck and M. Lipkin), pp.71-100, Plenum Press, New York.

Temin, H.M. (1974). *Cancer Res.* 34, 2835-2941.

Thomas, L. (1959). *In* "Cellular and Humoral Aspects of the Hypersensitive State" (Ed. H.S. Lawrence), pp.529-532 Hoeber-Harper, New York.

Trosko, J.E. and Chu, E.H.Y. (1975). *Advanc. Cancer Res.* 21, 391-425.
Van Duuren, B.L. (1969). *Progr. Exp. Tumor Res.* 11, 31-68.
Van Duuren, B.L. and Melchionne, S. (1969). *Progr. Exp. Tumor Res.* 12, 55-94.
Watson, A.F. (1932). *Cancer Rev.* 7, 445-462.
Wattenberg, L.W. (1977). *Advanc. Cancer Res.* 26, 197-226.
Wattenberg, L.W. (1980). *J. Environm. Pathol. Toxicol.* 3, 35-52.
Weinstein, I.B., Lee, L.-S., Fisher, P.B., Mufson, A. and Yamasaki, H. (1979). *In* "Environmental Carcinogenesis" (Eds. P. Emmelot and E. Kriek), pp.265-285. Elsevier North Holland Biomedical Press, Amsterdam.
Welsch, C.W. and Aylsworth, C.F. (1983). *J. Natl. Cancer Inot.* 70, 215-221.
Woglom, W.H. (1926). *Arch. Pathol.* 2, 533-576 and 709-752.

CHEMICAL CARCINOGENESIS IN THE DEVELOPING
NERVOUS SYSTEM

M.F. Rajewsky

*Institut für Zellbiologie (Tumorforschung),
Universität Essen (GH) Hofelandstrasse 55, D-4300 Essen 1
Federal Republic of Germany*

INTRODUCTION AND GENERAL CONSIDERATIONS

With most of the known chemical carcinogens, initiation of the
multi-step process of carcinogenesis involves structural alterations of DNA in the respective target cells (Lawley, 1976;
Pegg, 1977; Weinstein, 1977; Grover, 1979; Pullman *et al.*,
1980; Rajewsky, 1980a). In general, covalent binding occurs
between nucleophilic centres (electron-rich N and O atoms) in
cellular DNA and highly reactive, electrophilic derivatives
("ultimate carcinogens") generated from the respective parent
compounds ("pre-carcinogens") either enzymatically or via non-
enzymatic decomposition (Miller and Miller, 1976; 1979). The
accessibility of nucleophilic sites in DNA is to a certain
extent dependent on the degree of DNA packing, i.e. on chromatin structure (Nehls and Rajewsky, 1981a,b). Most DNA-reactive
chemical carcinogens have also been shown to be mutagenic
(McCann *et al.*, 1975; Nagao *et al.*, 1978; Hollstein *et al.*,
1979). The positive correlation of carcinogenicity and mutagenicity does not, however, constitute proof for an obligatory
requirement of mutation (nor even of modifications of DNA
structure in general) for malignant transformation, since
cellular macromolecules other than DNA also contain multiple
nucleophilic sites which react with carcinogen-generated
electrophiles. Nevertheless, the central importance of DNA
structure and conformation for the expression of genetic information provides a strong argument for a critical role of
DNA alterations in the initiation of malignant transformation.
    Structural modifications of DNA by chemical carcinogens may

THEORIES AND MODELS
IN CELLULAR TRANSFORMATION

lead to local alterations of nucleotide sequence (mutations)
and helical distortions, and in certain cases facilitate the
transition of the B-form of the double helix to a left-handed
Z-conformation (Wang *et al.*, 1979; Sage and Leng, 1980; Möller
et al., 1981; Santella *et al.*, 1981). Carcinogen-modified DNA
components could, however, also affect the precision of DNA
rearrangements (transpositional events in the genome may often
be associated with normal development/differentiation), cause
inappropriate rearrangements and amplification of genes as
well as chromosome translocations and deletions, and interfere
with the patterns of mRNA processing (splicing) and of DNA
methylation (Crick, 1979; Lapeyre and Becker, 1979; Rajewsky,
1980a; Cairns, 1981; Ehrlich and Wang, 1981; Fuchs *et al.*,
1981; Lavi, 1981; Riggs and Jones, 1983; Rowley, 1983). The
common denominator of all these mechanisms is an interference
with the genetic programmes of target cells. Therefore, more
information is needed on the molecular basis of eucaryotic
gene expression, on the mechanisms controlling phenotypic
differentiation and cell proliferation in developing and
mature cell systems, and on the particular genes involved in
these processes. The wide spectrum of differing tumour cell
phenotypes observed in mammals may not merely reflect the
expression of different combinations of genes characteristic
of the phenotypes of the corresponding normal cells of origin
in the course of development and differentiation of the respective cell lineages, it could also indicate that qualitat-
ively different phenotypic shifts may share the property of
resulting in a malignant behaviour of specific types of cells
in their respective tissue environment. The recent successful
use of the DNA transfection approach (Hayward *et al.*, 1981; Lane
et al., 1981; Weiberg, 1981; Reddy *et al.*, 1982; Tabin *et al.*,
1982; Land *et al.*, 1983; Newbold and Overell, 1983; Ruley, 1983)
has opened the way for a more detailed characterization of normal
or structurally altered cellular genes ("c-onc genes"), or of
their viral homologues ("v onc genes") introduced into the cellular genome, whose inappropriate expression is associated with
malignant transformation (Bishop, 1983). It will be most important, although not an easy task, to define the respective
gene products and their precise role in relation to the structure and function of normal and malignant cells (Müller and Verma,
1984).

The later stages of the maturation of cells to a terminally
differentiated state are generally accompanied by a cessation
of proliferative activity. In mature cells, the nonproliferative state can either be of an apparently irreversible nature
(e.g. in mature neurons or granulocytes), or be reversible
("G_0-cells") under special physiological conditions, such as
the requirement for reparative or functional hyperplasia (e.g.
in hepatocytes or hormonally controlled cell systems).

Temporary nonproliferative states of part of a cell population
are, however, also characteristic of stem cells, and probably
of committed precursor cells at more advanced stages of maturation (Rajewsky, 1972; Lajtha, 1979; Holtzer *et al.*, 1981).
   Like UV-induced photoproducts in DNA (Hanawalt *et al.*. 1979),
certain carcinogen-DNA adducts can be specifically recognized,
removed, and repaired by cellular enzymes (Rajewsky *et al.*,
1977; Margison and O'Connor, 1979; Lehmann and Karran, 1981;
Seeberg and Kleppe, 1981; Lindahl, 1982). Enzyme systems responsible for the recognition and elimination of critical DNA
lesions appear to be differentially expressed in different
cell types, tissues and species. Statistically, most persistent
(i.e. non-repaired) carcinogen-DNA adducts are localized in
transcriptionally silent parts of the genome. They become effective only when the functional integrity of the respective DNA sequences is put to the test in the course of gene activation
(by further progression of cells along the developmental/
differentiation pathway; by the induction of cells to express
previously inactive genes; or by triggering cells to enter the
cell cycle from a G_o-state, e.g. by the action of tumour promoters). It appears that malignant conversion occurs much
more readily, if not exclusively, after exposure of cells to
carcinogenic agents during earlier, proliferation-linked
stages of their differentiation pathway (or during a prolifer-
ation-competent G_o-state) than in target cells that have reached
a terminally differentiated, irreversibly nonproliferative state.
Therefore, the question is of particular interest, whether
along the differentiation pathway of a given cell lineage,
specific stem cell and precursor cell stages can be defined
where the gene programme can be shifted to the expression of
a malignant phenotype with higher than random probability
(Rajewsky *et al.*, 1977; Rajewsky, 1980b).
   Molecular and cellular mechanisms underlying the multi-
stage process of malignant transformation and tumorigenesis
can be particularly well studied in so-called "pulse-carcino-
genesis systems"; i.e. in systems where, after a single dose
of a short-lived carcinogen sufficient to produce a high
tumorigenic effect, the process proceeds autonomously without
the complication of continued interaction of the target cell
population(s) with the carcinogen. In such systems the process of carcinogenesis can be separated operationally into
three phases: phase A, period of carcinogen interaction with
target cells ("initiation"); phase B, time interval between
phase A and phase C; and phase C, period of tumour growth,
beginning with the onset of (clonal) proliferation of tumorigenic cells. In spite of its crucial importance, least is
presently known about phase B which often constitutes the
longest of the three phases and appears to encompass a sequence

of phenotypic changes (including acquisition of the capacity
for continuous proliferation) in the cells which ultimately
become tumorigenic (Laerum and Rajewsky, 1975; Barrett and
Ts'o, 1978; Kakunaga et al., 1980). During phase B, tumour
promoters can exert their effects (i.e. modify gene expression
and induce cell proliferation in the target cell population,
see Berenblum, 1975; Hecker et al., 1982). Probably of great
importance, but as yet largely unexplored, are the various
kinds of controlling influences (via short-range and long-
range humoral signals or cell-cell interactions) exerted during
phase B upon the potential tumorigenic cells by their particular tissue environment. Such microenvironmental influences
may represent an important element of control and variation
in the process of carcinogenesis. They are likely to be dependent on maturation- and age-related changes in the host
organism as well as on its genetic constitution, and on temporary reactions of the host to non-physiological factors.
In this context it should not be overlooked that the majority
of cells in a particular target tissue or cell system, although not undergoing tumorigenic conversion, are nevertheless
subject to the initial interaction with the carcinogen. This
may lead to disturbances of the normal, precisely balanced
control of cell proliferation and expression of cellular phenotypes, and of cell population structure and tissue architecture,
thereby influencing the transition probability of "initiated"
cells to the ultimate tumorigenic state. In target cell systems capable of reparative hyperplasia, chemical carcinogens
generally cause a dose-dependent increase in the rate of cell
proliferation due to their cytotoxic-effects (Rajewsky,
1967, 1972). An increased rate of reparative proliferation
of parenchymal liver cells, resulting from partial surgical
elimination of part of this cell population, has been shown
to enhance the hepatocarcinogenic effect of chemical carcinogens (Craddock, 1975).

Among the various classes of tumorigenic chemicals, the
alkylating N-nitroso-carcinogens have probably been characterized best with respect to their reaction products in DNA
(Lawley, 1976; Pegg, 1977; Grover, 1979; O'Connor et al.,
1979; Singer, 1979; Rajewsky, 1980a). These agents include
the alkylnitrosamines (which require bioactivation by cellular enzymes) and the alkylnitrosoureas and alkylnitro-
nitrosoguanidines (which undergo rapid, non-enzymatic decomposition in vivo). The resulting electrophilic alkyl
substituents are small in comparison with the bulky adducts
formed by reaction of DNA with carcinogenic hydrocarbons or
aromatic amines. A typical representative of the carcinogenic
alkylnitrosoureas is ethylnitrosourea, EtNU (Ivankovic and

Druckrey, 1968). EtNU has become a model carcinogen for the
study of mechanisms underlying both the tissue (cell type)-
tropism of the carcinogenic effect and its dependence on the
developmental(differentiation) stage of the target cells at the
time of carcinogen-exposure (Rajewsky, 1977, 1980b, 1982,
1983).

CARCINOGENESIS BY ETHYLNITROSOUREA (EtNU) IN THE RAT

Tissue (Cell Type)- Tropism of the Carcinogenic Effect

EtNU undergoes rapid (half-life, < 8 minutes) non-enzymatic
decomposition *in vivo*, thereby generating a highly reactive
ethyldiazonium ion (Goth and Rajewsky, 1972). When EtNU is
systemically applied to experimental animals, nucleophilic
sites in cellular macromolecules become ethylated to a similar
extent in all tissues, as shown by radiochromatographic analyses of rat DNA following injection of radiolabelled EtNU (Goth
and Rajewsky, 1974a,b) or by radioimmunoassay (Müller and
Rajewsky, 1978, 1980, 1983a). In spite of the similar initial
degree of ethylation in all tissues, a single pulse of EtNU
applied to foetal or newborn rats of the inbred BDIX strain
(Druckrey, 1971) results predominantly in malignant neuroectodermal neoplasms, while tumours in tissues other than the
brain and peripheral nervous systems (PNS) are rarely detected
(neural tissue-tropism of the carcinogenic effect). The yield
of neuroectodermal tumours and the latency period are dose-
dependent (Druckrey *et al.*, 1970b; Rajewsky *et al.*, 1977) and
strain-dependent (Druckrey *et al.*, 1970a). Following trans-
placental pulse-exposure to EtNU and subsequent transfer to a
long-term culture system, foetal BDIX-rat brain cells undergo
malignant transformation *in vitro* after a time period similar
to the time required for tumour formation *in vivo* after the
same carcinogen dose (Laerum and Rajewsky, 1975; Rajewsky *et
al.*, 1977; Laerum *et al.*, 1979).

Developmental(Differentiation) Stage-Dependence of the Carcino-
genic Effect

The neuroectodermal tumorigenicity of EtNU is strongly dependent on the developmental stage of the nervous system at the
time of carcinogen exposure. Being highest after an EtNU-
pulse during late prenatal and early postnatal development,
the tumorigenic effect decreases strongly in animals exposed
to the same dose of EtNU at a later age, in accordance with
the rapidly decreasing proportion of proliferative immature
neural target cells in the postnatal brain and PNS (Rajewsky *et al.*,

1977; Rajewsky, 1982, 1983). The carcinogenic effect is thus
inversely correlated with the developmental (differentiation)
stage of the neural cell populations, and appears to require the
presence of proliferative neural precursor cells at the time of
carcinogen exposure. However, tumorigenicity also decreases
when the EtNU pulse is applied at developmental stages prior
to prenatal day 15, and no neuroectodermal tumours were observed (in limited numbers of experimental animals) after exposure to EtNU before prenatal day 11 (Ivankovic and Druckrey,
1968). At the latter developmental stage, the total number of
cells in BDIX-rat brain (almost all proliferating) reaches a
value of approximately 10^5 (Müller and Rajewsky, 1983a); i.e.
in 20 rat embroys exposed to EtNU on prenatal day 11, the integral number of neural target cells would amount to $\sim 2 \times 10^6$.
    A number of studies indicate that the developmental period
of maximum sensitivity in terms of the neuro-oncogenic effect
of EtNU varies in different species. Thus, only a low incidence of neural tumours has been observed in several mouse
strains after late prenatal or neonatal administration of EtNU
(Denlinger et al., 1974; Jones et al., 1976). Postnatal application of EtNU to Mongolian gerbils has resulted in malignant
tumours originating from (neural crest-derived) cutaneous
melanocytes but not in tumours of the brain or PNS (Kleihues
et al., 1978). On the other hand, Stutman (1979) observed
mainly brain tumours (besides some kidney and ovarian tumours)
when immunologically competent (nu/+) or incompetent (nu/nu)
CBA/H or BALB/c mice were treated with EtNU on day 12-14 of
prenatal development, while after treatment on day 16-18 most
tumours were found in lung, liver (males) and kidney. Similar
findings were reported for rabbits, where EtNU caused predominantly neural tumours when applied during early prenatal
development, whereas exposure to EtNU during later foetal
stages led mainly to kidney tumours (Stavrou et al., 1975,
1977; Fox et al., 1975). Careful analyses are, therefore,
required in order to specify phases of increased carcinogenic
risk during development/differentiation of a given cell system
in different species.

Quantification of Alkylation Products in DNA by Radiochroma-tography and Immunoanalysis

The detection and quantification of alkylation products in
the DNA of target tissues and cells require highly sensitive
analytical methods. Radiochromatographic techniques (Baird,
1979), although used most extensively in the past, are limited
in their sensitivity mainly by the specific radioactivity of
the respective $[^3H]$- or $[^{14}C]$-labelled carcinogens. Under
favourable conditions, one alkylated base can be detected in

∿ 10^6 molecules of the corresponding normal base, and relatively large amounts of DNA (i.e. large numbers of cells) are
necessary for analysis. With the exception of recently developed ^{32}P "post-labelling" techniques (Randerath *et al.*, 1981;
Gupta *et al.*, 1982), radiochromatography requires the use of
radioactively labelled (i.e. laboratory-synthesized) carcinogens. Hence, the detection of specific carcinogen-DNA adducts
in (e.g. human) tissues and cells exposed to low doses of non-
radioactive (e.g. environmental) agents is not possible. This
situation has been improved by the recent development of immuno-
analytical procedures, using high-affinity polyclonal and monoclonal antibodies (antibody affinity constants, 10^9 to > 10^{10}
l/mol) directed against specific alkylation products in DNA
(Rajewsky *et al.*, 1980; Müller and Rajewsky, 1981; Adamkiewicz
et al., 1982; Müller *at al.*, 1982). Using a competitive radioimmunoassay (RIA) developed by Müller and Rajewsky (1978, 1980)
for the detection of 0^6-ethyldeoxyguanosine 0^6-EtdGuo) in DNA,
0^6-EtdGuo can be quantified at an 0^6-EtdGuo/deoxyguanosine
molar ratio of ∿ 3 x 10^{-7} in a hydrolysate of 100 μg of ethylated DNA (corresponding to the DNA content of ∿ 10^7 diploid
cells). This detection limit is lowered even further when
alkyladeoxynucleosides to be quantified are separated from the
DNA hydrolysate by high performance liquid chromatography
prior to the RIA. Monoclonal antibodies are now available for
the specific detection of different DNA alkylation products
and their spectrum is being further expanded (Adamkiewicz *et
al.*, 1982). Furthermore, the application of monoclonal antibodies has now been extended to their use in immunostaining
techniques for the detection and quantification of DNA alkylation products both in the nuclei of individual cells by
immunofluorescence (Adamkiewicz *et al.*, 1983), and in isolated
DNA molecules by immune electron microscopy (Nehls *et al.*,
1984).

Distribution of Ethylation Products in Chromosomal DNA

About a dozen different ethylation products are formed in DNA
exposed to EtNU (Loveless, 1969; Lawley, 1976; Singer *et al.*,
1978; O'Connor *et al.*, 1979; Singer, 1979; Rajewsky, 1980a).
The following products are formed by ethylation on oxygen
atoms (∿ 80% of all ethylation products of DNA): 0^6-EtdGuo
(∿ 10%), 0^2-ethyldeoxythymidine (0^2-EtdThd; ∿ 7%), 0^2-
ethyldeoxycytidine (0^2-EtdCyd; ∿ 4%), 0^4-ethyldeoxythymidine
(0^4-EtdThd; ∿ 3%) and ethylphosphotriesters (∿ 56%). Products resulting from ethylation on nitrogen atoms in DNA are:
7-ethyldeoxyguanosine (7-EtdGuo; ∿ 14%), 3-ethyldeoxyadenosine
(3-EtdAdo; ∿ 5%) 7-ethyldeoxyadenosine (7-EtdAdo; ∿ 0.4%),
1-ethyldeoxyadenosine (1-EtdAdo; ∿ 0.3%), 3-ethyldeoxycytidine

(3-EtdCyd; $\sim$ 0.2%), 3-ethyldeoxyguanosine (3-EtdGuo; $\sim$ 0.1%) and 3-ethyldeoxythymidine (3-EtdThd; $\sim$ 0.1%).

In the case of the ethylation products O^6-EtdGuo, O^2-EtdCyd, O^4-EtdThd, 3-EtdThd, 3-EtdCyd and 1-EtdAdo the alkyl groups are localized on atoms normally involved in Watson-Crick base pairing. The relative overall frequencies of these ethylation products in DNA are the same, regardless of whether the reaction with EtNU occurs *in vivo*, in cell cultures or with purified DNA *in vitro* (Goth and Rajewsky, 1974a,b; Singer *et al.*, 1978). However, recent measurements on individual DNA molecules using monoclonal anti-(O^6-EtdGuo) antibodies in conjunction with immune electron microscopy, indicate a strongly non-random distribution along DNA at least of this ethyldeoxynucleoside (Nehls *et al.*, 1984). The relative O^6-EtdGuo content in DNA has also been determined in chromatin of different folding levels, isolated from foetal rat brain cells and briefly exposed to EtNU *in vitro* (Nehls and Rajewsky, 1981a,b). By RIA for O^6-EtdGuo, it was shown that compared with naked DNA (relative value, 1.0), the degree of O^6-deoxyguanosine ethylation decreases from the DNA of extended (histone H1-free) chromatin fibres ($\sim$0.6) to the DNA in nucleosomes (core particles; $\sim$ 0.5), and is lowest in the DNA of condensed chromatin fibres ("superbeads", Renz *et al.*, 1977; $\sim$ 0.4). Independent of the chromatin folding level, nucleophilic sites located in the major and minor groove, and in base-pairing regions of the DNA double helix, appear to be equally accessible to the reactive ethyldiazonium ion. Furthermore, fractions of chromosomal DNA which are preferentially digested with DNase 1 (transcribable conformation, Garel and Axel, 1976; Weintraub and Groudine, 1976), were found to have a higher initial O^6-EdtGuo content than chromosomal DNA less susceptible to this enzyme (i.e. non-transcribable genome regions).

The carcinogenicity of different alkylating N-nitroso carcinogens is positively correlated with their relative extent of alkylation on oxygen atoms (e.g., O^6-EtdGuo) as compared to nitrogen atoms (e.g., 7-EtdGuo) in DNA (O'Connor *et al.*, 1979). For example the initial O^6-EtdGuo/7-EtdGuo ratio in DNA is $0.6 - 0.7$ for the potent carcinogen EtNU (Goth and Rajewsky, 1974b; Singer *et al.*, 1978), while for the weakly carcinogenic diethylsulfate this ratio is $\sim$ 0.003 (Sun and Singer, 1975). The relative extent of oxygen alkylation in DNA is a function of the type of reaction mechanism characteristic of the respective agent. Thus, a bimolecular nucleophilic (SN2) reaction will lead to an O/N alkylation ratio lower than that resulting from an SN2 mechanism with a tendency towards a unimolecular (SN1) reaction (Ingold, 1953; Lawley, 1976).

Differential Enzymatic Removal of Alkylation Products from DNA in Different Tissues and Types of Cells

The initial degree of ethylation by EtNU in the DNA of pre-natal ($\geq$ 11th day of gestation; Müller and Rajewsky, 1983a) or early postnatal rat brain (Goth and Rajewsky, 1974a,b) is not significantly different from that found in the DNA of adult brain and other "low carcinogenic risk" tissues (Goth and Rajewsky, 1972, 1974a,b). However, as shown by kinetic anal-yses after a pulse of EtNU to prenatal ($\geq$ 11th day of gesta-tion) or postnatal BDIX-rats, O^6-EtdGuo is rapidly removed from liver DNA (and less rapidly from the DNA of other tissues) but very slowly from brain DNA (Goth and Rajewsky, 1974a,b; Müller and Rajewsky, 1983a). Analyses in other rat strains (BDIV, Fisher), have given the same results (Rajewsky *et al.*, 1977; Chang *et al.*, 1980). The difference in the elimination rate of O^6-EtdGuo from brain versus liver DNA is so large that a specific enzymatic recognition and elimination mechanism had to be assumed for this particular ethylation product (Goth and Rajewsky, 1974a,b; Rajewsky *et al.*, 1977). In contrast to O^6-EdtGuo, other ethyldeoxypurines such as 3-EtdAdo and 7-Etd Guo are eliminated from the DNA of brain and other rat tissues at much faster rates than does O^6-EtdGuo from brain DNA. In-deed, with the exception of O^6-EtdGuo, large differences in tissue-specific elimination rates are not apparent for any alkylation product thus far investigated (including O^4-EtdThd; Müller and Rajewsky, 1983b). The persistence of O^6-EtdGuo in brain DNA, and the high rate of DNA replication of neural pre-cursor cells during the transformation-sensitive period of brain development, may thus be important factors contributing to the neural tissue-tropism of the carcinogenic effect of EtNU in the rat. O^6-EtdTuo not eliminated from DNA like O^4-EtdThd (Abbott and Saffhill, 1977), miscodes in DNA replication and transcription (Loveless, 1969; Abbott and Saffhill, 1977, 1979). The comparatively high extent of oxygen alkylation in DNA by EtNU appears to be responsible for the remarkable potency of this agent as a point mutagen in eukaryotic systems (Russel *et al.*, 1979; Vogel and Natarajan, 1979a,b; Johnson and Lewis, 1981). However, genetic consequences other than point mutations could equally result from structural modifi-cations persisting in DNA, and may be equally or even more relevant to malignant transformation (see Introduction and General Considerations, Müller and Rajewsky, 1983b).

When plotted semilogarithmically, the kinetics of the elimination of O^6-EtdGuo from cellular DNA generally appear to be bi- (or multi-) componential. Several mechanisms, alone or in combination, could account for this phenomenon: (1) an (O^6-EtdGuo)-removing enzyme (or (one of) several

enzymes), synthesized at relatively low rate, is initially
present in excess and consumed upon reaction; (2) O^6-EtdGuo is
differentially accessible in the DNA of chromatin of different
folding levels (see above); and (3) the tissue is composed of
subpopulations of cells with different capacities for enzymatic elimination of O^6-EtdGuo. Considerable efforts have been
made to identify and characterize the enzyme(s) responsible
for the removal of O^6-alkylguanine and other alkylation products from cellular DNA. Thus, DNA glycosylases have been
found in bacteria and mammalian cells that remove 3-alkyl-
adenine and 7-alkylguanine from DNA (Laval *et al.*, 1981;
Margison and Pegg, 1981; Singer and Brent, 1981; Lindahl,
1982). An "adaptive response" has been discovered in *E. coli*
which is inducible by low concentrations of simple methylating
agents (Samson and Cairns, 1977; Jeggo *et al.*, 1977), and involve the transfer and binding of a methyl group from the O^6
of guanine in DNA to a cysteine residue in an acceptor protein which is thereby inactivated (Karran *et al.*, 1979; Foote
et al., 1980; Olsson and Lindahl, 1980). The acceptor protein
thus has the properties of a DNA methyltransferase. Similar
O^6-methylguanine-DNA methyltransferase activities capable of
transferring methyl and, less efficiently, ethyl groups from
the O^6 of guanine in DNA to cysteine residues in the acceptor
proteins, have recently been isolated from mouse and rat liver
(Bogden *et al.*, 1981; Mehta *et al.*, 1981; Pegg *et al.*, 1983)
and in human lymphoid cells (Harris *et al.*, 1983). An active
protein fraction specifically reducing the O^6-alkylguanine
content of alkylated DNA *in vitro* had previously been isolated
from rodent and human liver homogenates (Pegg and Hui, 1978;
Pegg and Balog, 1979; Pegg *et al.*, 1982). Furthermore, evidence has been obtained indicating that the enzyme system reducing the O^6-methylguanine content of DNA in rat liver has
an elevated activity during the S-phase (and possibly the
G_2/M-phase) of the cell cycle as compared to the G_1-phase and
to the G_0-state (Rabes *et al.*, 1979; Pegg *et al.*, 1981). The
enzymatic elimination of O^6-alklguanine from liver DNA is less
efficient after high carcinogen doses ("saturation" of the
enzyme system; Kleihues and Margison, 1976). In different
species this saturation effect occurs at different carcinogen
dose levels. For example, the liver of the Syrian golden
hamster has a much lower saturation threshold than rat liver
(Margison *et al.*, 1976; Stumpf *et al.*, 1979; Montesano, 1982).
Correspondingly, hamster liver is sensitive to the induction
of hepatocellular cancer by a single dose of dimethylnitros-
amine for example, but rat liver is not (Tomatis and Cefis,
1967). It is not clear whether, in addition to the apparently
constitutive O^6-alkylguanine eliminating enzyme activity,
there is also an inducible response in mammalian systems,

analogous to the "adaptive response" in *E. coli*. An elevated
elimination capacity has been observed in rat liver in response to pretreatment with low doses of dialkylnitrosamines,
1.2-dimethylhydrazine, N-acetylaminofluorene, and 3,3-dimethyl-
1-phenyltriazene (see Montesano, 1981). However, the observed
relatively low increase in elimination activity would also be
compatible with an increased fraction of proliferating hepatocytes in S-phase, i.e. regenerative hyperplasia in response to
the cytotoxic pretreatment (Rajewsky, 1967, 1972).

The important question of cell type- and developmental/
differentiation stage-dependent differences in the capacity
for enzymatic elimination of critical alkylation products from
DNA has not yet been investigated, except for the case of
parenchymal versus non-parenchymal rat liver cells after treatment with 1,2-dimethylhydrazine (Lewis and Swenberg, 1980).
This agent induced hemangiosarcomas but not hepatocellular
carcinomas in rats, and O^6-methylguanine was shown to accumulate selectively in the DNA of non-parenchymal cells. In the
future this approach will be facilitated considerably by the
use of anti-alkyldeoxynucleoside monoclonal antibodies, for
example in conjunction with sensitive immunostaining procedures (Adamkiewicz *et al.*, 1983). Moreover, these techniques
will permit the study of enzymatic repair processes in small
amounts of cells, such as during prenatal stages of development or in bioptic tissue samples. In the EtNU-rat brain system, it will be important to investigate whether during early
prenatal stages (prior to day 11-12 of gestation) the enzyme
activity responsible for the elimination of O^6-EtdGuo from
neural precursor cells is equally low or higher than during
later pre- and postnatal development (Müller and Rajewsky,
1983a), and whether the DNA repair capacity of neural cells
varies as a function of cell type and stage of development
(differentiation).

In conclusion, the formation of specifically structured,
persistent carcinogen-DNA adducts (e.g. O^6-alkylguanine) may
play an important role in the initiation of the process of
carcinogenesis, and (via mechanisms which remain to be clari-
fied) may lead to, or facilitate, those alterations in the
cellular genome that ultimately result in the expression of
malignant phenotypes. Methods for the sensitive detection
and quantitation of specific carcinogen-DNA adducts in cells
exposed to non-radioactive (e.g. environmental) carcinogens
have considerable relevance for the identification of DNA
damage and for the characterization of cellular repair capacity. Enzyme systems for the specific recognition, elimination, and repair of critical DNA lesions appear to be differentially expressed in different cell types, tissues and
species. The capacity of cells to repair carcinogen-modified

DNA may thus constitute one of the determinants for the probability of malignant transformation, no less important than the expression of enzymes required for the metabolic activation of many carcinogens to their ultimate reactive forms. Under conditions of an equal degree of initial carcinogen-target cell interaction, the probability of tumorigenic conversion may vary with the type and differentiation state of the target cells; i.e. within multicomponential cell systems subpopulations of cells may be identified that are characterized by an elevated risk of malignant transformation (with the possible further complication that different "high risk" cell types and differentiation stages may be found for different types of carcinogens).

ACKNOWLEDGEMENTS

Experimental studies in the author's laboratory were supported by the Deutsche Forschungsgemeinschaft (SFB 102, A1 and A9), by the Commission of the European Communities (ENV-544-D[B]), and by the Ministerium für Wissenschaft und Forschung Nordrhein-Westfalen (II B5-Fa 8758).

REFERENCES

Abbott, P.J. and Saffhill, R. (1977). *Nucleic Acids Res.* 4, 761-769.

Abbott, P.J. and Saffhill, R. (1979). *Biochim. Biophys. Acta* 562, 61-61.

Adamkiewicz, J., Drosdziok, W., Eberhardt, W., Langenberg, U. and Rajewsky, M.F. (1982). *In* "Indicators of Genotoxic Exposure" (Eds. B.A. Bridges, B.E. Butterworth and I.B. Weinstein). Banbury Report 13, pp.265-276. Cold Spring Harbor Laboratory, Cold Spring Harbor, New York.

Adamkiewicz, J., Ahrens, O., Huh, N. and Rajewsky, M.F. (1983). *J. Cancer Res. Clin. Oncol.* 105, A15.

Baird, W.M. (1979). *In* "Chemical Carcinogens and DNA" (Ed. P.L. Grover), pp.59-83. CRC Press, Boca Raton.

Barrett, J.C. and Ts'o, P.O.P. (1978). *Proc. Natl. Acad. Sci. USA* 75, 3761-3765.

Berenblum, I. (1975). *In* "Cancer: A Comprehensive Treatise", Vol.1, (Ed. F.F. Becker), pp.323-344. Plenum Press, New York.

Bishop, J.M. (1983). *Ann. Rev. Biochem.* 52, 301-354.

Bogden, J.M., Eastman, A. and Bresnick, E. (1981). *Nucleic Acids Res.* 9, 3089-3102.

Cairns, J. (1981). *Nature (Lond.)* 289, 353-357.

Chang, M.J.W., Hart, R.W. and Koestner, A. (1980). *Cancer Lett.* 9, 199-205.

Craddock, V.M. (1975). *Chem.-Biol. Interact.* 10, 313-321.

Crick, F. (1979). *Science* 204, 264-271.

Denlinger, R.H., Koestner, A. and Wechsler, W. (1974). *Int. J. Cancer* 13, 559-571.

Druckrey, H. (1971). *Arzneim.-Forsch.* 21, 1274-1278.

Druckrey, H., Landschütz, C. and Ivankovic, S. (1970a). *Z. Krebsforsch.* 73, 371-386.

Druckrey, H., Schagen, B. and Ivankovic, S. (1970b). *Z. Krebsforsch.* 74, 141-161.

Ehrlich, M. and Wang, R.Y.-H. (1981). *Science* 212, 1350-1357.

Foote, R.S., Mitra, S. and Pal, B.C. (1980). *Biochem. Biophys. Res. Comm.* 97, 654-659.

Fox, R.R., Diwan, B.A. and Meier, H. (1975). *J. Natl. Cancer Inst.* 54, 1439-1448.

Fuchs, R.P.P., Schwartz, N. and Daune, M.P. (1981). *Nature (Lond.)* 294, 657-659.

Garel, A. and Axel, R. (1976). *Proc. Natl. Acad. Sci. USA* 73, 3966-3970.

Goth, R. and Rajewsky, M.F. (1972). *Cancer Res.* 32, 1501-1505.

Goth, R. and Rajewsky, M.F. (1974a). *Proc. Natl. Acad. Sci. USA* 71, 639-653.

Goth, R. and Rajewsky, M.F. (1974b). *Z. Krebsforsch.* 82, 37-64.

Grover, P.L. (1979). "Chemical Carcinogens and DNA", Vol.I and II. CRC Press, Boca Raton.

Gupta, R.C., Reddy, M.V. and Randerath, K. (1982). *Carcinogenesis* 3, 1081-1092.

Hanawalt, P.C., Cooper, P.K., Ganesan, A.K. and Smith, C.A. (1979). *Annu. Rev. Biochem.* 48, 783-836.

Harris, A.L., Karran, P. and Lindahl, T. (1983). *Cancer Res.* 43, 3247-3252.

Hayward, W.S., Neel, B.G. and Astrin, S.M. (1981). *Nature (Lond.)* 290, 475-480.

Hecker, E., Fusenig, N.E., Kunz, W., Marks, F. and Thielmann, H.W. (1982). "Carcinogenesis. A Comprehensive Survey, Vol.7, Co-carcinogenesis and Biological Effects of Tumour Promoters". Raven Press, New York.

Hollstein, M., McCann, J. and Angelosanto, F.A. (1979). *Mutat. Res.* 65, 133-226.

Holtzer, H., Pacifi, M., Croop, J., Boettinger, D., Toyama, Y., Payette, R., Biehl, J., Dlugosz, A. and Holtzer, S. (1981). *Fortschr. Zool.* 26, 207-225.

Ingold, C.K. (1953). "Structure and Mechanism in Organic Chemistry". Cornell University Press, Ithaca, New York.

Ivankovic, S. and Druckrey, H. (1968). *Z. Krebsforsch* 71, 320-360.

Jeggo, P., Defais, M., Samson, L. and Schendel, P. (1977). *Mol. Gen. Genet.* 157, 1-9.

Johnson, F.M. and Lewis, S.E. (1981). *Proc. Natl. Acad. Sci.*
    USA 78, 3138-3141.
Jones, E.L., Searle, C.E. and Smith, T.W. (1976). *Acta*
    Neuropathol. 36, 57-70.
Kakunaga, T., Lo, K.-Y., Leavitt, J. and Ikenaga, M. (1980).
    In "Carcinogenesis; Fundamental Mechanisms and Environ-
    mental Effects" (Eds. B. Pullman, P.O.P. Ts'o and H. Gelboin),
    pp.527-541. Reidel, Dordrecht-Boston-London.
Karran, P., Lindahl, T. and Griffin, B. (1979). *Nature (Lond.)*
    280, 76-77.
Kleihues, P. and Margison, G.P. (1976). *Nature (Lond.)*259,
    153-155.
Kleihues, P., Bücheler, J. and Riede, U.N. (1978). *J. Natl.*
    Cancer Inst. 61, 458-863.
Laerum, O.D. and Rajewsky, M.F. (1975). *J. Natl. Cancer*
    Inst. 55, 1177-1187.
Laerum, O.D., Haugen, Å. and Rajewsky, M.F. (1979). *In*
    "Neoplastic Transformation in Differentiated Epithelial
    Cell Systems *in vitro*" (Eds. L.M. Franks and C.B. Wigley),
    pp.190-201. Academic Press, London, New York.
Lajtha, L. (1979). *Differentiation* 14, 23-34.
Land, H., Parada, L.F. and Weinberg, R.A. (1983). *Nature*
    (Lond.) 304, 596-602.
Lane, M.-A., Sainten, A. and Cooper, G.M. (1981). *Proc. Natl.*
    Acad. Sci. USA 78, 5158-5189.
Lapeyre, J.N. and Becker, F.F. (1979). *Biochem. Biophys. Res.*
    Comm. 87, 698-705.
Laval, J., Pierre, J. and Laval, F. (1981). *Proc. Natl. Acad.*
    Sci. USA 78, 852-855.
Lavi, S. (1981). *Proc. Natl. Acad. Sci. USA* 78, 6144-6148.
Lawley, P.D. (1976). *In* "Chemical Carcinogens" (Ed. C.E.
    Searle). ACS Monograph No.173, pp.83-244. American Chem-
    ical Society, Washington, D.C.
Lehmann, A.R. and Karran, P. (1981). *Int. Rev. Cytol.* 72,
    101-146.
Lewis, J.G. and Swenberg, J.A. (1980). *Nature (Lond.)* 288,
    185-187.
Lindahl, T. (1982). *Annu. Rev. Biochem.* 51, 59-85.
Loveless, A. (1969). *Nature (Lond.)* 223, 206-207.
Margison, G.P. and O'Connor, P.J. (1979). *In* "Chemical
    Carcinogens and DNA" Vol.1 (Ed. P.L. Grover), pp.111-159.
    CRC Press, Boca Raton.
Margison, G.P. and Pegg, A.E. (1981). *Proc. Natl. Acad. Sci.*
    USA 78, 861-865.
Margison, G.P., Margison, J.M. and Montesano, R. (1976).
    Biochem. J. 157, 627-634.
McCann, J., Choi, E., Yamasaki, E. and Ames, B.N. (1975).
    Proc. Natl. Acad. Sci. USA 72, 5135-5139.

Mehta, J.R., Ludlum, D.B., Renard, A. and Verly, W.G. (1981). *Natl. Acad. Sci. USA* 78, 6766-6770.

Miller, E.C. and Miller, J.A. (1976). *In* "Chemical Carcinogens" Ed. C.E. Searle). ACS Monograph 174, pp.737-762. American Chemical Society, Washington, D.C.

Miller, J.A. and Miller, E.C. (1979). *In* "Environmental Carcinogenesis" (Eds. P. Emmelot and E. Krieh), pp.25-50. Elsevier North-Holland Biomedical Press, Amsterdam.

Möller, A., Nordheim, A., Nichols, R.S. and Rich, A. (1981). *Proc. Natl. Acad. Sci. USA* 78, 4777-4781.

Montesano, R. (1982). *J. Supramolec. Struct. Cell Biochem.* 17, 259-273.

Müller, R. and Verma. I. M. (1984). *Curr. Top. Microbiol. Immunol.* 112, 73-115.

Müller, R. and Rajewsky, M.F. (1978). *Z. Naturforsch.* 33c, 897-901.

Müller, R. and Rajewsky, M.F. (1980). *Cancer Res.* 40, 887-896.

Müller, R. and Rajewsky, M.F. (1981). *J. Cancer Res. Clin. Oncol.* 102, 99-113.

Müller, R. and Rajewsky, M.F. (1983a). *Cancer Res.* 43, 2897-2904.

Müller, R. and Rajewsky, M.F. (1983b). *Z. Naturforsch.* 38c, 1023-1029

Müller, R., Adamkiewicz, J. and Rajewsky, M.F. (1982). *In* "Host Factors in Human Carcinogenesis" (Eds. H. Bartsch and B. Armstrong). IARC Scientific Publications No.39, pp.463-479.

Nagao, M., Sugimura, T. and Matsushima, T. (1978), *Annu. Rev. Genet.* 12, 117-159.

Nehls, P. and Rajewsky, M.F. (1981a). *J. Cancer Res. Clin. Oncol.* 99, A38.

Nehls, P. and Rajewsky, M.F. (1981b). *Europ. J. Cell Biol.* 24, 17.

Nehls, P., Rajewsky, M.F., Spiess, E. and Werner, D. (1984). *EMBO J.* 3, 327-332.

Newbold, R.F. and Overell, R.W. (1983). *Nature (Lond.)* 304, 648-651.

O'Connor, P., Saffhill, R. and Margison, G.P. (1979). *In* "Environmental Carcinogenesis" (Eds. P. Emmelot and E. Kriek), pp.73-96. Elsevier/North Holland Biomedical Press, Amsterdam.

Olsson, M. and Lindahl, T. (1980). *J. Biol. Chem.* 255, 10569-10572.

Pegg, A.E. (1977). *Adv. Cancer Res.* 25, 195-269.

Pegg, A.E. and Balog, B. (1979). *Cancer Res.* 39, 5003-5009.

Pegg, A.E. and Hui, G. (1978). *Biochem. J.* 173, 739-748.

Pegg, A.E., Perry, W. and Bennett, R.A. (1981). *Biochem. J.*

__197__, 195_201.
Pegg, A.E., Roberfroid, M., Van Bahr, C., Foote, R.S., Mitra,
   S., Brésil, H., Likhachev, A. and Montesano, R. (1982).
   Proc. Natl. Acad. Sci. USA __79__, 5162-5165.
Pegg, A.E., Wiest, L., Foote, R.S., Mitra, S. and Perry, W.
   (1983). *J. Biol. Chem.* __258__, 2327-2333.
Pullman, B., Ts'o, P.O.P. and Gelboin, H. (1980). "Carcino-
   genesis: Fundamental Mechanisms and Environmental Effects"
   Reidel, Dordrecht, Boston, London.
Rabes, H.M., Kerler, R., Wilhelm, R., Rode, G. and Riess, H.
   (1979). *Cancer Res.* __39__, 4228-4236.
Rajewsky, M.F. (1967). *Europ. J. Cancer* __3__, 335-342.
Rajewsky, M.F. (1972). *Z. Krebsforsch.* __78__, 12-30.

Rajewsky, M.F. (1980a). *In* "Molecular and Cellular Aspects
   of Carcinogen Screening Tests" (Eds. R. Montesano, H.
   Bartsch and L. Tomatis). IARC Scientific Publications No.
   27, pp.41-54. International Agency for Research on Cancer,
   Lyon.
Rajewsky, M.F. (1980b). *Arch. Toxicol.* Suppl. 3, 229-236.
Rajewsky, M.F. (1982). *In* "Chemical Carcinogenesis" (Ed. C.
   Nicolini), pp.363-379. Plenum Press, New York.
Rajewsky, M.F. (1983). *Recent Results in Cancer Res.* __84__, 63-
   76.
Rajewsky, M.F., Augenlicht, L.H., Biessmann, H., Goth, R.,
   Hülser, D.F., Laerum, O.D. and Lomakina, L.Ya. (1977). *In*
   "Origins of Human Cancer" (Eds. H.H. Hiatt, J.D. Watson
   and J.A. Winsten), pp.709-726. Cold Spring Harbor Labor-
   atory, Cold Spring Harbor, New York.
Rajewsky, M.F., Müller, R., Adamkiewicz, J. and Drosdziok, W.
   (1980). *In* "Carcinogenesis: Fundamental Mechanisms and
   Environmental Effects" (Eds. B. Pullman, P.O.P. Ts'o and
   H. Gelboin), pp.207-218. Reidel, Dordrecht, Boston, London.
Randerath, K., Reddy, M.V. and Gupta, R.C. (1981). *Proc.
   Natl. Acad. Sci. USA* __78__, 6126-6129.
Reddy, P.E., Reynolds, R.K., Santos, E. and Barbacid, M.
   (1982). *Nature (Lond.)* __300__, 149-252.
Renz, M., Nehls, P. and Hozier, J. (1977). *Proc. Natl. Acad.
   Sci. USA* __74__, 1879-1883.
Riggs, A.D. and Jones, P.A. (1983). *Adv. Cancer Res.* __40__,
   1-30.
Rowley, J.D. (1983). *Nature (Lond.)* __301__, 290-291.
Ruley, H.E. (1983). *Nature (Lond.)* __304__, 602-606.
Russell, W.L., Kelly, E.M., Hunsicker, P.R., Bangham, J.W.,
   Maddux, S.C. and Phipps, E.L. (1979). *Proc. Natl. Acad.
   Sci. USA* __76__, 5818-5819.
Sage, E. and Leng, M. (1980). *Proc. Natl. Acad. Sci. USA*
   __77__, 4597-4601.

Samson, L. and Cairns, J. (1977). *Nature (Lond.)* 267, 281-283.

Santella, R.M., Grunberger, D., Weinstein, I.B. and Rich, A. (1981). *Proc. Natl. Acad. Sci. USA* 78, 1451-1455.

Seeberg, E. and Kleppe, E. (1981). "Chromosome Damage and Repair". Plenum Press, New York.

Singer, B. (1979). *J. Natl. Cancer Inst.* 62, 1329-1339.

Singer, B. and Brent, T.P. (1981). *Proc. Natl. Acad. Sci. USA* 78, 856-860.

Singer, B., Bodell, W.J., Cleaver, J.E., Thomas, E.H., Rajewsky, M.F. and Thon, W. (1978). *Nature (Lond.)* 276, 85-88.

Stavrou, D., Hänichem, T. and Wriedt-Lübbe, I. (1975). *Z. Krebsforsch.* 84, 207-215.

Stavrou, D., Dahme, E. and Schröder, B. (1977). *Z. Krebsforsch.* 89, 331-339.

Stumpf, R., Margison, G.P., Montesano, R. and Pegg, A.E. (1979). *Cancer Res.* 39, 50-54.

Stutman, O. (1979). *Path. Res. Pract.* 165, 170.

Sun, L. and Singer, B. (1975). *Biochemistry* 14, 1795-1802.

Tabin, C.J., Bradley, S.M., Bargmann, C.I., Weinberg, R.A., Papageorge, A.G., Scolnick, E.M., Dhar, R., Lowy, D.R. and Chang, E.H. (1982). *Nature (Lond.)* 300, 143-149.

Tomatis, L. and Cefis, F. (1967). *Tumori* 53, 447-452.

Vogel, E. and Natarajan, A.T. (1979a). *Mutat. Res.* 62, 51-100.

Vogel, E. and Natarajan, A.G. (1979b). *Mutat. Res.* 62, 101-123.

Wang, A.H., Quigley, G.J., Kolpak, F.J., Cranford, J.L., Van Boom, J.A., Van der Macel, G. and Rich, A. (1979). *Nature (Lond.)* 282, 680-686.

Weinberg, R.A. (1981). *Biochim. Biophys. Acta* 651, 25-35.

Weinstein, I.B. (1977). *In* "Mechanismes d'Alteration et de Réparation du DNA, Relations avec la Mutagenèse et la Cancerogenèse Chimique. Colloques Internationaux du CNRS No.256" pp.2-40. Centre National de la Recherche Scientifique, Paris.

Weintraub, H. and Groudine, M. (1976). *Science* 193, 848-856.

Index